CELL-BASED BIOSENSORS

CELL-BASED BIOSENSORS

JAROSLAV RACEK

Head, Department of Clinical Biochemistry
University Hospital
Plzeň, Czech Republic

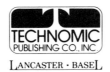

TECHNOMIC
PUBLISHING CO., INC.

LANCASTER · BASEL

Cell-Based Biosensors
a TECHNOMIC®publication

Published in the Western Hemisphere by
Technomic Publishing Company, Inc.
851 New Holland Avenue, Box 3535
Lancaster, Pennsylvania 17604 U.S.A.

Distributed in the Rest of the World by
Technomic Publishing AG
Missionsstrasse 44
CH-4055 Basel, Switzerland

Main entry under title:
  Cell-Based Biosensors

A Technomic Publishing Company book
Bibliography: p.
Includes index p. 105

Library of Congress Catalog Card No. 94-61808
ISBN No. 1-56676-190-5

CHAPTER 1

Introduction

Today we hear more and more about biosensors in connection with the analysis of biological material – especially in relation to their selectivity and their possibility of measuring the concentration of various substances (even in optically opaque media) after being immersed in reaction mixtures in bioreactors, or by introducing them into living organisms. Biosensors as analytical devices are composed of three main parts that are connected to each other and form an inseparable unit.

The first part – the *receptor* (recognition system) – is represented by a biomolecule isolated from living organisms such as enzymes, antibodies, lectines, hormone receptors, or nucleic acid fragments. The biomolecule is able to recognize the special substance selectively on the basis of their specific interaction. During this interaction a signal arises (the product of an enzyme reaction for instance), which is then registered by the second part of a biosensor – by the *transducer.* Ion-selective electrodes and field-effect transistors or thermistors can work as transducers, as can optical and other transducers. They usually produce an electrical signal that is amplified and registered by the third part of a biosensor.

The most common receptor that has been used is an enzyme molecule. This classic example of a receptor shows great selectivity for the substrate to be estimated. Among the various types of transducers, potentiometric or amperometric electrodes are used most often; they detect the fall of the substrate concentration or the rise of the product concentration. These parts form the device that is, according to its components, known as the enzyme electrode. Enzyme electrodes represent the most common type of biosensors. Many of them are commercially available and form a basis for most analyzers in the determination of blood glucose or lactate concentration.

In the mid-1970s it was found that not only enzymes, but also whole living microbial cells could be used for the biosensor preparation instead of an isolated enzyme; enzyme activity within microbial cells was used in this case. The first cell-based biosensor was the microbial electrode with the cells of *Acetobacter xylinum* immobilized in a cellulose membrane on the surface of an oxygen electrode. It was used for the determination of ethanol concentrations on the basis of the measurement of oxygen consumption during ethanol assimilation in bacterial cells [1]. In the following years lots of new microbial biosensors were described; they use the high activity of a specific enzyme within the cells of various bacterial and yeast strains. Later on, other forms of living cells were also applied to the biosensor construction; tissue slices from various organs of animals and higher plants, in connection with the appropriate transducer, form tissue biosensors.

The aim of this work is to acquaint the reader with the problems of the construction and use of cell-based biosensors. To understand these problems, it is necessary to know the functioning principles and properties of these biosensors; the most important is the selectivity. It is extremely significant to know the possibilities for improving the selectivity to such a degree that the cell-based biosensors could be used in analytical praxis.

CHAPTER 2

Cell-Based Biosensors

2.1 COMPARISON OF CELL-BASED AND ENZYME BIOSENSORS

Cell-based biosensors are analytical devices; the connection of suitable cells as a receptor with a transducer is the principle of cell-based biosensors. As previously mentioned, the high enzyme activity within the cells is usually used; the enzyme catalyzes the conversion of a determined substrate, and the transducer responds to the resulting product with a change of its signal, which is then registered by means of a special electronic attachment. The function of most cell-based biosensors is thus, in many features, analogical with that of biosensors with immobilized isolated enzymes. In spite of it, the use of whole cells has some advantages in comparison with enzyme biosensors:

- Isolation, purification, and immobilization of enzymes are often very difficult; they can be omitted.
- Some enzymes can lose their activity during isolation or immobilization if this process leads to the damage of the active center or to the disintegration of enzyme complexes; this risk is also eliminated by the use of the whole cells.
- Enzymes in the cell's natural environment are usually extremely stable.
- Multi-step enzyme reactions in intact cells can be used, making it possible to avoid the preparation of complicated artificial multi-enzyme systems.
- Coenzymes and activators are often present in the cells, and thus, it

3

is not necessary to add them into the system; the cell itself usually cares for their effective regeneration.

• Other principles of measurement can be used, namely those based on observation of respiratory activity of living cells and its alteration due to the presence of a detected substance.

• Cultivation of microbial cells, or preparation of tissue slices in the laboratory, is easy and cheap when compared with the preparation of a pure enzyme.

It can be said that the cell represents the most suitable milieu for en-zymes – they are "naturally immobilized" within the cell – and that is why they are marked by a great stability.

Despite all positive features, the use of whole cells for preparation of biosensors has also some disadvantages:

• The reaction can run more slowly because the substrate must get over the cell membrane on its way to the enzyme, as well as the product on its way from the cell to the transducer. Some substrates, especially macromolecular compounds, cannot be used for this reason.

• Other metabolic pathways in the cells can be the source of the side products that are also registered by a transducer; this leads to the decrease of the biosensor selectivity if those cells are used for its preparation.

These properties, especially the problem of the biosensor selectivity and the possibilities of its improvement, will be discussed in detail in Chapters 5 and 6.

2.2 TYPES OF CELL-BASED BIOSENSORS

2.2.1 Classification According to the Type of Cells Used

Various types of cells can be used for the biosensor construction. The most common are bacterial or yeast cells; then we speak about *microbial biosensors*. In other cases, however, multicellular organisms can also be used. Thus, biosensors with immobilized mould mycelium [2], a slice of a fruit-body of the higher fungus [3], or with a paste prepared from lichens [4], were described. The cells of higher plants and animals, usually pre-pared from the appropriate organ in the form of a thin slice, are present on the transducer surface of *tissue biosensors* [5,6]. And finally, we can find the biosensors based on human erythrocytes. These blood corpuscles rep-

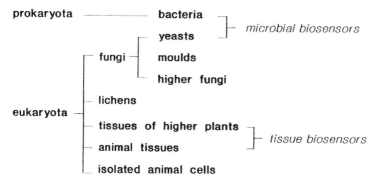

FIGURE 2.1. Cell types used for preparation of cell-based biosensors.

resent a specialized animal tissue that is not rigid and that comes in the form of isolated cells known from microbial biosensors [7–9]. Besides erythrocytes, there are also other isolated animal cells that can be used for a biosensor construction—for example, leucocytes or fibroblasts [10]. Figure 2.1 shows the biosensor classification according to the cells used for their construction.

It is necessary to mention two peculiarities:

(1) The use of two different cell types on the surface of one transducer is the first peculiarity. These cells can catalyze two reactions that are linked to each other. The substrate of the first reaction is the analyzed substance, and the product of the second reaction is registered by a transducer [11]. In another case, the second type of cells is able to amplify the measured signal in a process of enzyme cyclization [12].

(2) The second peculiarity is the coimmobilization of an isolated enzyme and whole cells on the transducer surface. The function of this so-called *hybrid biosensor* resembles the coimmobilization of the two cell types already described [6,13]. Some hybrid biosensors even work on the basis of three enzyme reactions linked to each other. The first reaction is catalyzed by an isolated enzyme, and the next two take place in two different kinds of bacterial cells [14,15].

2.2.2 Classification According to the Relation of the Cells to the Transducer

According to the relation of the cells to the transducer we can distinguish two kinds of biosensors [Figure 2.2(a) and 2.2(b)]: membrane and reactor. *Membrane biosensors* have the biocatalyzer in the form of a membrane

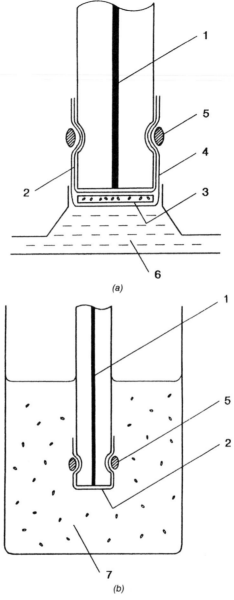

FIGURE 2.2. (a) Membrane biosensor and (b) Reactor biosensor, both with an oxygen electrode as a transducer; 1—platinum cathode, 2—teflon membrane, 3—membrane with immobilized cells, 4—dialysis membrane, 5—rubber O-ring, 6—chamber with a sample, 7—cell suspension with a sample in a reaction vessel.

containing the cell suspension, or formed with a tissue slice that is retained on the transducer surface. The transducer can examine the reaction in its initial quick phase (initial reaction rate mode) or after the response reaches the constant value (steady-state mode). Most of the biosensors belong to this group of membrane biosensors. Their construction enables the repeated use of the biosensor without the necessity of membrane regeneration or replacement. In several cases, the plant tissue forms just a component of the electrode (transducer). This electrode type was prepared by mixing a paste or powder from a spinach leaf [16], ground beet root [17], or banana pulp [18,19], with graphite powder and liquid paraffin. The paste that was formed in the described way is usually placed in a glass capillary; it represents the electrode that can be used for amperometric or voltammetric detection of some substrates.

Reactor biosensors usually use a suspension of bacterial cells [19–24], or a suspension prepared from plant tissue [25], in a vessel reactor. The cells can also be immobilized on the bottom of the vessel, for example, in a polyacrylamide gel [26,27]. The transducer, such as a membrane potentiometric electrode, amperometric electrode, or a conductivity detector, is immersed into the cell suspension; in one case of a flow system, the transducer is even placed outside the reactor [22]. It can register the reaction from the very beginning [20,25], but in most cases the product is not estimated until the substrate is completely converted, which can take several hours. If the cells are not immobilized, it is necessary to renew the suspension after each measurement.

2.2.3 Classification According to the Transducer Type

The transducer is, in the majority of cases, represented by an ion-selective electrode that changes its potential according to the increase of the ion concentration due to the enzyme, which catalyzes the conversion of the measured substrate. The other possibility is an amperometric detection of substances that can be oxidized on an anode or reduced on a cathode. Potentiometric ion-selective electrodes introduce in the measurement a further selectivity factor—their response to one ion is stronger than to other ions. On the contrary, the use of amperometric detection always involves a danger of interference with other substances, especially those with a reducing effect that are often present in biological material in significant concentrations; their effect can be expressed in those cases when the electrode is plugged in as the anode. This problem will be discussed in greater detail in Section 5.1.3.

The voltammetric detection enables not only quantitative measurements, but also the differentiating of several electroactive compounds and, thus, the analysis of more than one compound at the same time. Related compounds can be quantified, and the signal of some interfering substances can also be easily subtracted [4,16,18,19].

Another possibility of electrochemical detection is represented by the use of ion-selective field-effect transistors (ISFET); it allows miniaturizing the biosensor size. This is important in the analysis of small volumes of biological material, and especially when the biosensors are to be used *in vivo* [28–31].

If the reaction products are ionizable, for example, in urea hydrolysis, an increase in conductivity can be measured [25]. The last type of transducer is a thermistor thermometer, which can register the heat production during the enzyme reaction [27]. The biosensors with this type of transducer show the worst selectivity, which on the other hand, can be an advantage in some special cases—see Section 6.19. The measurement of reaction heat is not used in practice very often; it requires a rather complicated apparatus that provides perfect heat isolation of the reactor with the cells.

2.3 PRINCIPLES OF CELL-BASED BIOSENSOR FUNCTIONING

2.3.1 Determination of Enzyme Reaction Product

The cell biosensors are, in most cases, based on the detection of the substances originating from the substrate in enzyme reactions within immobilized cells. The measured product can be ammonia, carbon dioxide, hydrogen ions, hydrogen peroxide, hydrogen sulfide, gaseous hydrogen, and, more rarely, other products. These products often arise in a one-step reaction, catalyzed with one enzyme. Some examples are enzyme deamination of adenosine in the mucosal cells of a mouse small intestine [32], glutamate decarboxylation in the microbial cells of *Escherichia coli* [33] or in a slice of yellow squash [34], or the splitting of β-lactam cycle of cephalosporins in the cells of *Citrobacter freundii* [35].

$$\text{adenosine} + H_2O \xrightarrow{\text{adenosine deaminase}} \text{inosine} + NH_3$$

$$\text{glutamate} \xrightarrow{\text{glutamate decarboxylase}} \text{4-aminobutyric acid} + CO_2$$

$$\beta\text{-lactam} + H_2O \xrightarrow{\text{cephalosporinase}} \text{acid } (H^+)$$

Other biosensors use a two-step reaction, catalyzed with two enzymes. This is the case of nitrate determination by the biosensor with *Azotobacter vinelandii* [36].

$$NO_3^- + NADH + H^+ \xrightarrow{\text{nitrate reductase}} NO_2^- + NAD^+ + H_2O$$

$$NO_2^- + 3NADH + 4H^+ \xrightarrow{\text{nitrite reductase}} NH_3 + 3NAD^+ + 2H_2O$$

When determining histidine, this substrate is transformed in the cells of the bacterial strain *Pseudomonas* in four reactions that are linked to each other; two ammonia molecules are liberated during this process [37]. That is why the determination of histidine with a microbial biosensor is more sensitive than the determination of histidine using the enzyme electrode with histidine-ammonia lyase, which catalyzes only the first from these reactions, and thus, results in the liberation of only one ammonia molecule [38].

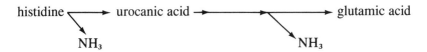

Cell-based biosensors of this type can also be used for the estimation of catalytic activity of enzymes if they are sensitive to the product that originates from a suitable substrate in an enzyme catalyzed reaction. Two biosensors for the estimation of α-amylase activity were described. The first of them is based on the detection of maltose by the cells of *Bacillus subtilis*, in which maltase synthesis was induced. The other hybrid biosensor contains glucoamylase and *Bacillus subtilis* in two membranes; the glycolytic metabolic pathway within the bacterial cells was induced [39]. The biosensor for the determination of proteases is based on the same microbe type. It responds to oligopeptides after the splitting of casein; the microbial cells are again specially prepared by cultivation in a peptide-rich medium [40].

In some cases, consumption of oxygen can be measured instead of measuring the increase of a product concentration. Some examples are: (1) the determination of phenol with the cells of *Trichosporon cutaneum* [41] or with a slice of a fruit-body of a fungus *Agaricus bisporus* [31], and (2) the use of biosensors with the cells of *Enterobacter agglomerans* [6] or a slice of yellow squash [6,42] for ascorbic acid determination. In these reactions oxygen takes part directly in the substrate conversion, and this type of biosensor must be differentiated from so-called respiratory electrodes; the principle of their functioning will be described in the next chapter.

Sometimes, it is more convenient to replace oxygen with another electron acceptor, as hexacyanoferrate(III) [2,7,43–46] or 2,6-dichlorphenolindophenol [47]. Then, we do not measure the fall in an oxygen partial pressure, but instead, we measure the oxidation of a reduced form of this artificial electron acceptor on the anode.

2.3.2 Examination of the Changes in Microbe Respiration

If microbial cells do not convert the substrate to a suitable product that could be measured with an ion-selective electrode, the microorganisms can be immobilized on the surface of an oxygen electrode. The electrode registers the respiratory activity of the cells as a fall in oxygen concentration near the cells. This type of biosensor, often called a *respiratory electrode,* was constructed for the determination of glucose and other sugars [48–50], ethanol [1,51], methanol [51,52], acetic acid [52,53], and other compounds. Since oxygen consumption is associated with production of carbon dioxide, the carbon dioxide gas-sensing electrode can also be used as a transducer [49].

Oxygen or carbon dioxide electrodes can estimate the assimilation of many various compounds; for this reason, this arrangement seems to be less specific, and the interference of many substances that are metabolizable in the microbial cells can be expected. This fact was used in the construction of biosensors for the estimation of water pollution with organic substances as biological oxygen demand (BOD); microbial cells that were cultivated in a rich medium and, thus, able to assimilate a broad spectrum of organic substances, are usually chosen for this purpose [26,54–59] – see also Section 6.19.

Another example of a respiratory electrode is that for the determination of vitamins – for example, thiamin. The increase in oxygen consumption as an expression of respiration of the yeast *Saccharomyces cerevisiae* in a membrane on the surface of an oxygen electrode is proportional to the concentration of this vitamin in the analyzed solution [60]. The respiratory electrode was also used to estimate the number of living cells in contaiminated food [61].

Respiratory electrodes have a wide spectrum of use in the determination of substances inhibiting microbial growth. Reduction of respiratory activity of microbial cells in this case becomes evident as a decrease in oxygen consumption or carbon dioxide production when compared with the blank. Biosensors with the cells of sensitive bacterial strains were used for the determination of tetracyclines [24], aminoglycoside antibiotics such as gentamicin [62,63], or nystatin and other polyene antimycotics [64,65]. This type of biosensor can be used for the detection of toxic substances in water and air; their function is based on the inhibition of respiratory processes in the cells of a sensitive microbe. The genetically deficient strain of *Bacillus subtilis* immobilized on the oxygen electrode was used for the screening of potential mutagens; they reduce the respiration of this strain, while the wild strain is not influenced by these substances — its cells are able to repair the damaged DNA-molecule [66]. Human foreskin fibroblasts or mouse leukemia cells placed on an oxygen electrode are sensitive bioreceptors for antitumor drugs [10].

Respiratory electrodes must use living cells exclusively, while the biosensors, based on the substrate conversion in one or several defined reactions, can also be constructed with dead cells. In order for quantitative results to be reached, the constant concentration of the cells in a suspension or in a membrane on the surface of a transducer must be guaranteed [24,61]. In addition, the cells must be in the same metabolic status; various phases of the microbe cultivation differ in the cells' respiration intensity [62,67]. Inhibition of microbial growth by the use of antibiotics, mutagens, or other toxic compounds is usually irreversible, and that is why in these cases the microbial suspension or membrane must be renewed after each measurement; the standard density and metabolic status of microbial cells must be strictly kept.

2.3.3 Determination of Released Intracellular Compounds

Some substances can cause the increase of cell membrane permeability or the lysis of the cells with the consequent release of intracellular components in the solution surrounding the cells [68,69]. The cells used for the determination of these substances are usually modified by a method that causes their cytoplasm to contain an atypical, naturally non-occurring ion, which is, after its release into extracellular space, detected with a proper ion-selective electrode.

Thus, the cells of a yeast *Saccharomyces cerevisiae*, containing cation Rb^+, were used for a quantitative estimation of nystatin; this antibiotic is the cause of Rb^+ release from the yeast cells [70].

The suspension of *Micrococcus lysodeicticus* intact cells, artificially loaded with a trimethylphenylammonium cation, serves for the determination of lysozyme in biological material. The cell membrane of this sensitive microbe is lysed by this enzyme, and the amount of the atypical cation released from the cells is proportional to lysozyme concentration in a sample [71].

2.3.4 Other Principles of Cell-Based Biosensor Functioning

The biosensor with thalli of various lichens in a graphite paste works on a different principle than all of the types of biosensors mentioned above. The predisposition for inorganic cation uptake by lichens from their substrates and from rainwater is used in this case. Heavy metal ions Pb^{2+}, Hg^{2+}, and Cu^{2+}, absorbed in a lichen component of the electrode, were differentiated and quantified voltammetrically. The electrode could be regenerated and reused [4].

The last example is represented by a biosensor for antidiuretic hormone determination. The biosensor is assembled by fitting a toad bladder over a sodium ion-selective electrode. The antidiuretic hormone influences the transport of sodium ions across the toad bladder in the direction to the Na^+-sensitive electrode; the change of its response depends on the hormone concetration in the analyzed solution [72].

CHAPTER 3

Construction and Peculiarities of Basic Types of Cell-Based Biosensors

3.1 MICROBIAL BIOSENSORS

It is necessary to obtain a suspension of suitable microorganisms (yeasts or bacteria) with sufficient activity of a special enzyme for microbial biosensor construction. This is usually achieved by cultivating microbial cells in a liquid medium containing the enzyme substrate that will be the estimated substance for the cell-based biosensor at the same time. The substrate induces enzyme synthesis within the cells. Since this procedure also influences the biosensor selectivity to the substrate, the problem of enzyme induction will be discussed in the chapter dealing with the selectivity enhancement of cell-based biosensors—see Section 6.8.

Native living cells are usually used for immobilization on the surface of a sensing electrode. Some researchers recommend increasing cell membrane permeability by, for example, (1) washing the cells in a hypotonic solution of complexone [74], (2) immersing them in a 40% solution of dimethylsulfoxide [2,44,46], or (3) even by destroying the cells with ultrasonic treatment [74–78]. These and other procedures not only facilitate a substrate diffusion to an intracellular enzyme, but sometimes they can be essential for good biosensor functioning and its selectivity—see Section 6.7. On the other hand, the cell damage can cause the impaired stability of the cell-based biosensor; the cells treated in this way cannot be used for the construction of respiratory electrodes.

Freeze-drying bacterial or yeast cells (besides influencing the cell membrane permeability) enables the long-term conservation of the cells with the high activity of a special enzyme, which was reached by the above-mentioned cultivation with the substrate. The lyophilized cells retain their enzyme activity at 4°C for several months. They can be used whenever desired for the reconstitution of the cell suspension suitable for the biosensor preparation [33,41,45–47,76,79].

If the reactor type of microbial biosensor is not used, an optimal process must be chosen for the retention of microbial cells near the transducer, which is usually on the measuring electrode surface. A semipermeable dialysis membrane is frequently used; it keeps the suspension, and it is fixed to the transducer by means of a rubber O-ring [2,36,37,41,45,60,75,79–88]. The use of various physical methods for the immobilization of microbial cells in a porous medium is another possibility. The membrane containing microbial cells is then held on the electrode surface again, with a semipermeable membrane for estimating polar compounds and, for example, with a teflon membrane to detect non-polar compounds. Microbial cells can be retained in an acetylcellulose membrane [6,46,51–54,89–96], collagen membrane [35,48,55,64], 2% agar gel [92,97], polyacrylamide gel [55,78], gelatin [96,97], filter paper [98], polyvinylalcohol [57], or polyvinylcaprolactam [29], or the cell suspension is applied in the mesh of a nylon net [8,33]. Sometimes this procedure is followed by membrane stabilization with glutaraldehyde [64,99,100]. Retention of the cells within calcium alginate [28,101] or kappa-carrageenan gel [10] is particularly convenient owing to its "cell-friendly" character. The method of cell immobilization and the character of the membrane that covers the cell layer influence the diffusion rate of the substrate and other substances to the cellls and transducer; therefore, they can determine such biosensor features as sensitivity, response time, and even selectivity to a special substrate.

If they are not used for measurements, microbial biosensors are usually stored in a refrigerator at +4°C with a tip immersed in a working buffer. Some researchers prefer the addition of the substrate into the buffer so that, in the case of immobilization of living cells, the nutrient supply would be ensured [36,90,94]. The biosensor stability can be very high in this case, even if it is stored at room temperature [102].

3.2 TISSUE BIOSENSORS

A slice of animal or plant tissue can be placed on the transducer surface if the tissue contains a high activity of the enzyme catalyzing conversion of the substrate that is to be detected. This so-called tissue electrode has, in comparison with microbial biosensors, several different features determining its advantages and disadvantages.

While bacteria or yeasts must first be cultured in a special liquid medium, it is very easy to prepare a tissue slice. Tissue is usually cut with a razor blade. It is necessary to choose and cut slices of a convenient thickness – usually within the range of 0.2–0.5 mm. It is difficult to prepare thinner slices, and enzyme activity in them may not be high enough; greater thickness causes a reduction in substrate diffusion rate, resulting in a long response time of the biosensor [34].

The tissue is usually fitted to the transducer with a semipermeable membrane [103–105]. In contrast to microbial biosensors, a nylon net can be used for this purpose: tissue integrity is usually great enough, and single cells cannot get loose from the tissue slice; at the same time, the nylon mesh is not a serious barrier for the substrate diffusion to the cells [5,106,107]. If the tissue slice is not firm enough, it is possible to improve it by cross-linking with albumin and glutaraldehyde [32,34,108]. A semipermeable dialysis membrane is usually used in these cases as well and is situated between the tissue slice and the transducer surface. The membrane protects the covering of the transducer surface with proteins and lipids from biological material.

The possibility of preparing a paste from the plant tissue and mixing it with a graphite powder and mineral oil to form a mass suitable for the construction of a proper measuring electrode was already discussed in Section 2.2.2. This is the case when a cell receptor and transducer are integrated into a single part.

When human erythrocytes are used as a biocatalyzer, the method of their immobilization resembles that of monocellular organisms [7,8].

Tissue slices can be stored for several months without reducing the activity of a special enzyme in the cells. The tissue is usually immersed in a buffer with the addition of a preservative that is necessary to guard against bacterial and mycotic contamination. Various substances can be used for this purpose, such as 0.002% chlorhexidine diacetate [34], 0.1% merthiolate [8,103], or sodium azide in concentrations of 0.02% [5,32,106,107–100] or 0.2% [103,110,111]. Ascorbate oxidase activity in a slice of yellow squash fruit retains its activity for at least one year when properly stored [42]. The same preservative is usually added to the buffer that is used between measurements; the biosensor tip with the tissue slice is immersed in it. Nevertheless, it is always necessary to test whether the preservative does not act as an enzyme inhibitor in the tissue.

By means of microbe cultivation in a liquid medium with a substrate addition, we can reach not only the activity increase of a proper enzyme, but also the improvement of a biosensor selectivity. This is not possible in the case of tissue biosensors. That is why it is necessary to choose tissue with a high enzyme activity carefully. When in 1979 the porcine kidney was first used for the construction of a tissue biosensor for glutamine determination, the favourable properties of this device were not a great surprise because the high glutaminase activity in tubular cells of the kidney had been well known for a long time [5]. The knowledge of metabolic processes in animal tissues enabled the construction of new tissue biosensors in following years. On the contrary, plant tissues were thought to be unsuitable for the biosensor construction, thanks to their slower metabolism and less specific biocatalytic activity. Nevertheless, it was found that growing portions of plants (such as leaves, root tips, fruits, and vegetables) that store nutrients for future growth and propagation can serve as a successful cell-based receptor. For this purpose, slices from the above-mentioned organs are used; leaves can even be used without any preparation; however, when they are applied for the estimation of hydrophilic compounds, the hydrophobic cuticula from the leaf surface must be removed [105]. The use of a paste prepared from a plant tissue is also quite common [16–19]. It is important to choose the appropriate part of a plant organ; for example, glutamate dehydrogenase and ascorbate oxidase activity in a squash mesocarp is several times higher than in other parts of the fruit [5,39]. The use of a tissue biosensor represents the only possibility in those cases when enzyme synthesis cannot be induced in the microbe cells, and we want to avoid the biosensor preparation with a purified enzyme.

In conclusion, we can summarize that—in comparison with microbial biosensors—tissue biosensors have an easier preparation, but their response time is usually longer due to a more difficult substrate diffusion.

3.3 HYBRID BIOSENSORS

As was previously stated, hybrid biosensors are analytical devices where two biocatalyzers are coimmobilized on the transducer surface—a purified enzyme and whole microbial cells, or a tissue slice with another active enzyme within the cells. Both enzymes catalyze the reactions that are linked with each other.

In general, it can be said that the isolated enzyme catalyzes the conversion of the estimated substrate into a metabolite of the cells [14,15,39,112,113], or on the contrary, the metabolic product of intact cells is (by a catalytic action of the isolated enzyme) transformed into the substance, which can be detected with an electrochemical transducer [21,114,116]. To ensure long-term stability of a hybrid biosensor, it is useful to stabilize the isolated enzyme with, for example, glutaraldehyde [14,15,39,114,115]; chemical linkage of enzyme molecules on the cell surface was also described [117]. As for the topical arrangement, two ways are possible: (1) the isolated enzyme and the cells form two separate membranes [14,15,39,114,115], or (2) enzyme molecules are dispersed among the cells [112,113,116,118]. Some hybrid biosensors are of a reactor type and use a sus-

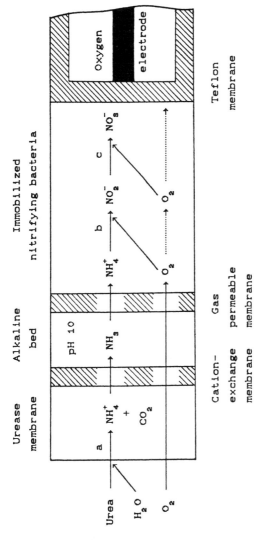

FIGURE 3.1. Principle of the hybrid urea biosensor with urease (a) and bacteria *Nitrosomonas sp.* (b) and *Nitrobacter sp.* (c). (Reprinted from Okada, T., I. Karube, and S. Suzuki: 1982. *Europ. J. Appl. Microbiol. Biotechnol.*, 14(3):149–154, with permission.)

pension of bacterial cells in a reactor vessel while the enzyme is placed in a membrane on the transducer surface.

The design of a hybrid biosensor for urea detemination is shown in Figure 3.1.

The construction of hybrid biosensors is more complicated than the construction of simple microbial or tissue biosensors; the laboriousness is usually compensated for with a higher selectivity that is demonstrated in the case of the urea hybrid electrode — see Section 6.15.

CHAPTER 4

Properties of Cell-Based Biosensors

4.1 PROPERTIES COMPARABLE WITH THOSE OF ENZYME BIOSENSORS

The functional principle of most cell-based biosensors is not different from that of enzyme biosensors. Therefore, it is logical that most properties in both biosensor types are comparable.

Sensitivity of the substrate estimation usually lies within the concentration range of $10^{-3}-10^{-4}$ mol/l; sometimes it is 10^{-5} mol/l [21,119–124], or even higher [6,16,42,78,96,97,104]. The sensitivity value, in most cases, is comparable with the concentration of many metabolites in biological material. If other properties, such as a quick response and a sufficient selectivity, are fulfilled, this sensitivity enables the cell-based biosensors to be used in the analysis of blood, urine, food, fermentation broths, etc.

Reproducibility, expressed as a variation coefficient, is usually less than 5% [22,51,78,81,94,125] and, thus, again comparable with that of other analytical methods including enzyme biosensors (e.g., in medical practice it agrees with requirements for the reproducibility of clinical laboratory methods).

Many researchers have compared the analysis by cell-based biosensors with the results obtained by other analytical methods, such as spectrophotometry, gas chromatography, polarography, or in the case of biological oxygen demand with a classical five-day method. Practically all experiments obtained comparable results; the mathematical implication of these results was represented by high correlation coefficients, many times above 0.95 – see also Chapter 7.

4.2 PROPERTIES DIFFERENT FROM THOSE OF ENZYME BIOSENSORS

Besides the conforming properties mentioned above, some differences can be found between cell-based and enzyme biosensors. Some of these differences make the cell-based biosensors more advantageous; the others, on the contrary, can limit their use. In this section, we will go through two of these properties – the response time and biosensor stability. The problems of the third property – the biosensor selectivity – are so extensive and important that special attention will be given to it in the following two chapters – see Chapters 5 and 6.

4.2.1 Response Time of Cell-Based Biosensors

The response time in a cell-based biosensor can be a little slower than in an analogical biosensor with an isolated enzyme because the substrate must get over a cell membrane on its way to the enzyme. This is especially true in the case of tissue biosensors, if a tissue slice is too thick. The cell membrane can even be impermeable for a special substrate; these cells cannot be used for the analysis of this substance until the cell membrane permeability is artificially increased. This procedure, based on differences in cell membrane permeability of vital and permeabilized cells for various substrates, can also be used for the selectivity enhancement of cell-based biosensors – see Section 6.7.

On the other hand, in many cases the extension of the biosensor response time is not very pronounced, and it is often not a rule. In most cell-based biosensors the steady state is obtained within 2–10 min. The features of the cells themselves and the thickness of a layer with immobilized cells, as well as the quality of a membrane covering the cells, and a transducer type, play their part in biosensor response time. In examining carbon dioxide production, it is found that the measurement is slower than if the same reaction is observed as a fall in oxygen concentration [49] or ammonia production [25,83,86]; a carbon dioxide gas-sensing electrode is known to be much slower in its response than either of the above-mentioned electrodes.

Sometimes, it is better to examine a reaction course in its initial phase, which enables a very quick result. It we waited until the steady state were reached, and if we then added the time necessary for the biosensor regeneration with a restitution of an original signal value, some types of cell-based biosensors would be too slow in their response, and therefore, from a practical point of view, unuseable.

4.2.2 Stability of Cell-Based Biosensors

Most cell-based biosensors have an outstanding stability, and the response value is unchanged even after several weeks. Some cell-based biosensors can be used for two or more months [8,40,101], in one case, even when the biosensor was stored at room temperature [102]. This is made possible due to good enzyme stabilization in the cells. If the biosensor is stored properly, that is, in a buffer with a nutrient, an increase in its response can be observed; immobilized vital cells can grow and multiply, and thus, the specific enzyme activity increases [90]. If the same enzyme is used in an isolated form and held on the transducer surface in the same way as the whole cells, the stability of this enzyme biosensor is usually markedly lower. For example, in glutamine determination with a biosensor with glutaminase held on the surface of an ammonia gas-sensing electrode by means of a semipermeable membrane, the biosensor is stable for one day only, while the same biosensor with bacterial cells of *Sarcina flava* can be used for twenty days, and the tissue glutamine biosensor with a slice of porcine kidney shows the best stability—thirty days [13]. Similarly the microbial biosensor for histidine determination keeps its original response for twenty-two days [37], while an analogic biosensor with histidine-ammonia lyase is useable only for a week [38]. Also, in a great number of other cases, the biosensor life-time is noticeably higher if cells are used as a receptor [87,91,107,108]. The life-time of enzyme biosensors could be improved by enzyme immobilization with chemical methods [6]; the construction of such a biosensor is, however, more complicated and expensive than in the use of the whole cells.

It is unquestioned that enzyme activity in the cells often falls slowly, even with optimal biosensor storage. But if the initial enzyme activity is great enough, the value of the biosensor response is limited with a substrate diffusion rate across the membrane covering the cell layer. The fall in the biosensor response value can be observed only after such an enzyme activity depression, when the substrate conversion rate becomes lower than its diffusion to the cells. In this case, the biosensor stability is only apparently caused by an unchangeable enzyme activity in the cells [45].

CHAPTER 5

Causes of Cell-Based Biosensor Unselectivity

5.1 COMMON CAUSES FOR ALL TYPES OF BIOSENSORS

In all of these cases, interference is not dependent on the presence of a cell structure as a receptor; substances that are found in analyzed samples influence either the substrate or the transducer, or they act with another mechanism. The same type of interference can also be observed in the biosensors, or in other analytical methods such as spectrophotometry, where the isolated enzyme is used instead of the whole cells.

5.1.1 Product of Enzyme Reaction Present in Analyzed Sample

If the measured product of an enzyme reaction were present at the same time in the sample to be analyzed, an apparently high analyte concentration would be found had this fact not been considered. This can appear often, especially in biological material. Furthermore, as the interfering substance concentration fluctuates sample by sample, it is necessary to remove it before the analysis or to try to eliminate its influence by the subtraction of the blank value.

Many biosensors use deaminating reactions, mostly by determination of various amino acids, with an ammonia gas-sensing electrode as a transducer. In the case of blood or urine analysis, ammonia concentration in a sample can significantly elevate the results. The concentration ratio of the measured substance and ammonia in biological material predetermines the interference degree. Thus, ammonia does not interfere with urea determination in blood serum because urea concentration in this liquid is two orders higher that that of ammonia [84,94]. On the contrary, concentration of some amino acids in serum can be close to that of ammonia.

Similarly, carbon dioxide (or hydrogencarbonates) in biological material can interfere if its production is examined with a carbon dioxide electrode. Carbon dioxide from the sample can also interfere with hydrogen sulfide determination in a cysteine biosensor with the cells of *Proteus morganii;* the gas-sensing electrode used in this case is twice as sensitive to carbon dioxide as to hydrogen sulfide [85].

5.1.2 Reaction of Interfering Substance with the Analyte

In this case, the interfering substance reacts with the substrate and, thus, causes a real drop in its concentration. For example, if we add ascorbic acid into the hydrogen peroxide solution, hydrogen peroxide is progressively reduced, and we find its lower concentration [126]. This interference type can be observed not only when the cell-based biosensor—for example, the biosensor with human erythrocytes—is used, but also in all other methods for hydrogen peroxide determination, including methods based on a principle other than that of biosensors.

Ascorbic acid can reduce not only the concentration of a determined substrate, but also the concentration of the product that is formed from it in the cells and should then be registered by a transducer. Thus, in the case of a "banana electrode" for dopamine determination, this substrate is transformed to dopamine quinone in the cells of banana pulp, and this product is then regisitered amperometrically on the cathode. When the sample contained ascorbic acid, which reduced a small portion of quinone, a 10–20% decrease in the biosensor response to dopamine was observed [19].

5.1.3 Influence of the Interfering Substance on the Transducer

The influence of the interfering substance on the transducer is caused by a transducer unselectivity to a measured substance. Thus, when using an ammonium-selective electrode for NH_4^+ detection, other monovalent cations such as Na^+ and K^+ interfere [127]. An electrode for hydrogen sulfide determination responds not only to this compound, but also to other gaseous substances of an acid nature, for example, to carbon dioxide [85].

Many reductive substances can interfere with amperometric detection of an enzyme reaction product during its oxidation on the anode. The measured product is usually hydrogen peroxide; this product can be found in inorganic phosphate determination by a hybrid biosensor [114], and in oxalate determination by a tissue electrode using a ground beet root [17] or a banana skin [15], which are rich in oxalate oxidase. Another substance that can be oxidized on the anode is the reduced form of electron transfer mediators that are often used in reactions catalyzed by some oxidoreduc-

TABLE 5.1. Effect of Some Reducing Substances (1 mmol/l) on the Yeast Biosensor with Hansenula anomala *Compared with the Response of the Same Sensor without Yeast Cells.*

	Electrode Response in μA		
	Yeast Cells		
	Living	Inactivated	No Biocatalyst
Cysteine	0.162	0.153	0.160
Glutathione	0.156	0.158	0.158
Ascorbic acid	0.415	0.445	0.352
Uric acid	0.327	0.347	0.352
Lactate	0.622	0	0

Reprinted from Racek, J. and J. Musil. 1987. *Clin. Chim. Acta,* 167(1):59–65. With permission.)

tases: (1) hexacyanoferrate (II) in lactate [7,45–47,76], glucose [2], and ethanol biosensors [41] or (2) a reduced form of 2,6-dichlorphenolindophenol in lactate [47] and steroid determinations [128]. If the analyzed samples contain other substances with a reducing action, they can be oxidized on the anode; their oxidation results in a higher current and, thus, in an increased result. The interference degree depends neither on the presence of cells on the transducer surface nor on the enzyme activity within the cells (Table 5.1).

5.1.4 Enzyme Unselectivity for Determined Substrate

Most enzymes are strictly selective with respect to their substrate. Nevertheless, we can find some cases when one enzyme can also convert other substrates that differ only in their substituents or in the length of their carbon chains. At other times, the enzyme molecule can have an effect on the compounds with a specific bond. If we use this enzyme for substrate analysis, it is clear that we will estimate the sum of all substances transformed by the enzyme. Individual reaction rates, and thus, the biosensor sensitivity to these substances can vary even in the conversion of very similar substrates. Of course, this interference type is not characteristic for cell-based biosensors and can be observed in any analytical use of these less specific enzymes.

For example, the biosensor for tryptophane determination is based on the use of tryptophanase in bacterial cells of *Escherichia coli*. This enzyme splits off ammonia not only from tryptophane, but also from serine and cysteine, which interfere with tryptophane determination by this microbial biosensor [90]. Ascorbate oxidase also catalyses oxidation of isoascorbic acid; this compound interferes with vitamin C determination by both cell-based biosensors—with *Enterobacter agglomerans* [6] and a cucumber or yellow squash tissue slice [6,42]. Cysteine determination with a bacterial biosensor is based on L-cysteine dehydrogenase in bacterium *Proteus morganii*. This enzyme also splits off hydrogen sulfide from other sulfur amino acids, for example, from homocysteine [85].

All antibiotics of a cephalosporin group can be hydrolyzed by cephalosporinase. The biosensor based on this enzyme activity in the cells of *Citrobacter freundii* can therefore be used for analysis of various cephalosporin drugs [35]. The biosensor with the cells of *Nocardia opaca* uses steroid-Δ^1-dehydrogenase, the substrate of which are all 3-keto-4-ene-steroids. This biosensor responds to a number of steroid hormones—testosterone, cortisol, and androstenedione—certainly with unequal intensity [128].

The biosensor with the cells of *Arthrobacter nicotiana* responds to various free fatty acids because of its oxidation in the bacterial cells. The response degree rises with the length of the carbon chain from acetic acid (C_2) to caprylic acid (C_{10}) with the following quick decrease of sensitivity; palmitic and stearic acids give a negligible response (Figure 5.1). This sensitivity decrease can be explained as follows: the cells on the oxygen elec-

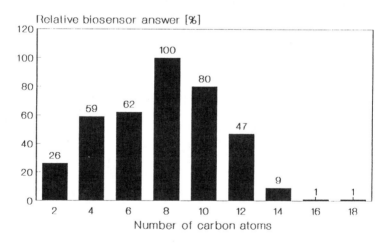

FIGURE 5.1. Relative sensitivity of the microbial biosensor with *Arthrobacter nicotiana* to saturated fatty acids in dependence on the length of their carbon chain; response to caprylic acid equals 100%. (Reprinted from Ukeda, H., G. Wagner, U. Bilitewski, and R. D. Schmid. © 1992. American Chemical Society, *J. Agr. Food. Chem.*, 40(11):2324–2327. With permission.)

trode surface are covered with a dialysis membrane that is impermeable for hydrophobic long-chain fatty acids [129].

The use of the biosensor with a sugar beet root slice for tyrosine determination is based on oxidation of this amino acid by tyrosinase. This enzyme is not very selective, and catalyses oxidation of a great number of phenolic substances, which interfere with different intensities [104]. On the contrary, the tyrosine biosensor with bacterium *Aeromonas phenologenes* uses intracellular tyrosine-phenol lyase resulting in ammonia detection; phenols do not interfere with this reaction, but another type of interference can be observed [81].

Also, other biosensors based on intracellular activity of monophenol oxidase or polyphenol oxidase are not entirely specific. They are (1) biosensors with a yeast *Trichosporon cutaneum* [41] or a slice of a fungal fruitbody *Agaricus bisporus* [3] for phenol determination, (2) catecholamine biosensors based on a spinach leaf [130] or banana pulp [19], and (3) a biosensor based on an eggplant fruit pulp that is senstitive to catechol [131]. Response intensities of some of the above-mentioned biosensors to phenolic compounds are summarized in Table 5.2. Unselectivity of phenoloxidases and different reaction rates in the oxidation of individual phenolic compounds according to the enzyme source can be seen from this comparison.

Similar to a substrate unspecificity, one enzyme can have a number of inhibitors. Thus, the hybrid biosensor for phosphate determination is based on the inhibitory action of this anion on acid phosphatase activity in a potato slice. Phosphates, fluorides, molybdates, and nitrates inhibit this enzyme, and they can be considered as interferants [114,115,188].

Finally, a different example is the determination of glucose or fructose with a biosensor based on permeabilized cells of *Zymmomonas mobilis*. The active enzyme in this bacterium is glucose-fructose oxidoreductase, which needs both of these sugars in equimolar amounts for its activity. Consequently, this biosensor can be used for the determination of either glucose or fructose, but only when the other one of these monosaccharides is present in a given amount [100].

5.1.5 Interference of Other Substrates of the Metabolic Pathway Used

The biosensors belonging to this group are based on a multi-step substrate transformation; the measured substance is produced or consumed only in some of the final reactions. That means that the whole metabolic pathway within the cells is necessary for the substrate determination. That is why all intermediates of the substrate transformation cause the same

TABLE 5.2. Phenol Biosensor with a Mushroom Slice, Dopamine Biosensor with a Banana Pulp, Tyrosine Biosensor with a Sugar Beet Root, and Catechol Biosensor with an Eggplant Fruit—Relative Response to Other Phenolic Compounds of the Same Concentration.

Mushroom Slice		Banana Pulp		Sugar Beet Root		Eggplant Fruit	
				Biosensor Response in %			
Phenol	100	Dopamine	100	Tyrosine	100	Catechol	100
Catechol	100	Catechol	100	3,4-Dihydroxy-phenylalanine	35	Dopamine	59
p-Cresol	94	Hydroquinone	94	2,4-Dichlorphenol	35	3,4-Dihydroxy-phenylalanine	13
p-Chlorphenol	90	Norepinephrine	90	p-Chlorphenol	12	Epinephrine	0
Pyrogallol	45	3,4-Dihydroxy-phenylglycol	45	Phenol	3	Tyrosine	0
3,4-Dihydroxy-phenylalanine	39	Epinephrine	39	o-Cresol	1	Phenol	0

Adapted after References [3,19,104,131], with permission.

biosensor response as the substrate itself. If we wanted to determine the same substrate with an analogical enzyme biosensor, it would have to be constructed by coimmobilization of all enzymes of that metabolic pathway; aside from its tremendously laborious construction, this biosensor would show the same degree of unselectivity as the cell-based electrode.

In the following paragraphs, several examples of this interference type will be shown. Thus, in the histidine biosensor with the cells of *Pseudomonas sp.*, which is based on the liberation of two ammonia molecules in a four-step transformation within these microbial cells (see also Section 2.3.1), urocanic acid was an interferant, because it is the first intermediate in histidine metabolism [37]. The biosensor for the determination of nitrilotriacetic acid (NTA) uses a multi-enzymatic degradation of this substrate into glycerate in the cells of a bacterial species *Pseudomonas*. The response to glycine and serine was similar to that of NTA since these substances are intermediates in NTA metabolism before ammonia production in the next to the last reaction; only ammonia is registered by a transducer (Figure 5.2) [86].

Intermediate metabolites of the multi-enzyme oxidative pathway of tryptophane, such as L-kynurenine, anthranilic acid, or pyrocatechol, interfere in tryptophane determination with the biosensor using bacterial cells of *Pseudomonas fluorescens* [96]. The last example represents a nitrate biosensor based on the cells of *Azotobacter vinelandii*, immobilized on an ammonia gas-sensing electrode. Nitrates are reduced in a two-step reaction—first to nitrites and then to ammonia (see Section 2.3.1). Since nitrite is an intermediate in this reaction, the biosensor response to nitrite is similar to the biosensor response to nitrate [36].

5.2 CAUSES TYPICAL ONLY FOR CELL-BASED BIOSENSORS

Besides the enzymes that are necessary for substrate transformation, many other enzymes are usually present in the cells. These enzymes are the cause of the most important interference type that is characteristic only of cell-based biosensors. All substrates of these enzymes can interfere with the main substrate determination if they have the same reaction product. The more abundant the enzyme supply in the cells, the higher the interference risk. That is why it is necessary to choose the cells with the least possible amount of active metabolic pathways, while the required enzyme is present in high activity; human erythrocytes can provide such an example. The analogical enzyme biosensor, which uses only the activity of the enzyme necessary for the substrate transformation, would definitely not respond to interferants of this group, having its selectivity higher in this respect.

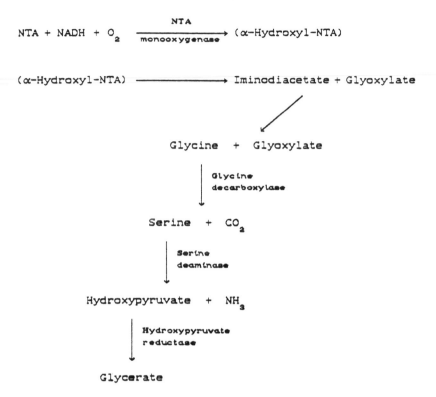

FIGURE 5.2. Metabolic pathway of nitrilotriacetic acid (NTA) degradation by *Pseudomonas sp.*

5.2.1 Presence of Other Enzymes Belonging to One Metabolic Pathway within the Cells

In many cases the substrate is converted into a measured product in a one-step enzyme reaction. If this is the final reaction of a metabolic pathway and if other enzymes belonging to this pathway are active within the cells, then all preceding intermediates are potentially interfering substances—the determined substrate will originate from them.

The biosensors for glutamate or aspartate determination with the cells of *Escherichia coli* or *Bacterium cadaveris* are good examples of the interference type described above. High activity of glutaminase or asparaginase can be found within the cells of these bacterial species. These enzymes catalyze conversion of glutamine to glutamate and asparagine to aspartate; that is why the glutamate biosensor also responds to glutamine [33], and the aspartate biosensor is sensitive not only to aspartate, but also to asparagine [87].

The same interference type can be observed in the case of some tissue biosensors. Thus, the tissue electrode for adenosine determination also responds to adenosine monophosphate (AMP) because of a high alkaline phosphatase activity in the cells of a mouse small intestine mucosa, which are used for the biosensor construction. This enzyme catalyzes the hydrolysis of AMP to adenosine and inorganic phosphate [32]. The guanine biosensor with a rabbit liver tissue is specific not only for this purine compound, but it also responds to guanosine. It is caused by guanosine phosphorylase in rabbit hepatocytes, which catalyzes guanosine conversion to guanine [103]. The biosensor with a slice of a rabbit muscle is sensitive to AMP and adenosine diphosphate, which can be metabolized to AMP in the muscle tissue [107].

5.2.2 Influence of Other Metabolic Pathways in the Cells

Numerous metabolic paths usually found in the cells are the cause of this interference type. It includes the generation of the measured product from a substrate other than the principal substrate; the signal registered by the electrode is usually increased. This interference in cell-based biosensors belongs to the most important types. In spite of trying to choose the microbe strain or the tissue with the lowest possible number of active metabolic paths and the highest activity of an appropriate enzyme (often increased by enzyme synthesis induction during cultivation in a substrate-rich medium), we can be surprised by the number and heterogeneity of interfering substances. It is not possible to mention all of the interfering substances in individual cell-based biosensors. We will try for a certain generalization, and in the end of this section several concrete examples of this interference type will be shown.

Glucose belongs to the most common energy sources for many microbes and tissues. Consequently, the expectation of its being a frequently interfering substance can be highly probable (Table 5.3). It is interesting that glucose also sometimes interferes in those cases where a transducer registers a substance that cannot originate from glucose—ammonia is an example. This phenomenon could be explained with the stimulation of the metabolism of nitrogen-containing substances in which ammonia is liberated [13,34].

It is always important to compare concentrations of the interfering substance, and the substrate that is to be determined in an analyzed sample, as in biological material. Thus, glucose interferes with lactate or cholesterol determinations in blood serum only if its concentration greatly exceeds the upper limit of the physiological range [78,132]. On the other hand, glucose in physiological concentrations can interfere with uric acid determination; the usual concentration of uric acid in blood serum is about

TABLE 5.3. Glucose Interference with Different Cell-Based Biosensors, Expressed as a Percentage of a Biosensor Response to Glucose; Biosensor Response to Its Main Substrate of the Same Concentration as That of Glucose Equals 100%.

Substrate	Cell Type	Measured Product	Interference Degree (%)	Ref.
Aspartame	*Bacillus subtilis*	O_2	300.0	[147]
Pyruvate	*Streptococcus faecium*	CO_2	51.3	[82]
Lactate	*Hansenula anomala*	O_2	22.2	[121]
Oxalate	Red beet root	H_2O_2	19.0	[17]
Urea	*Proteus mirabilis*	CO_2	9.4	[84]
Lactate	*Hansenula anomala*	$Fe(CN)_6^{4-}$	7.7	[132]
Histidine	*Pseudomonas sp.*	NH_3	5.5	[37]
Uric acid	*Pichia membranaefaciens*	CO_2	3.8	[133]
Cholesterol	*Nocardia erythropolis*	O_2	2.5	[78]
Glutamate	*Bacillus subtilis*	O_2	*	[144]
Glutamine	Porcine kidney	NH_3	*	[13]
Methylsulfate	*Hyphomicrobium sp.*	H^+	*	[79]
Phenol	*Trichosporon cutaneum*	O_2	*	[41]
Tryptophane	*Pseudomonas fluorescens*	O_2	*	[96]

*Interference described, not given quantitatively.

ten times lower than that of glucose, while concentrations of cholesterol or lactate in blood are of the same order as that of glucose [133].

Glucose is a strong interfering agent in hybrid biosensors for lactose [115], sucrose [134], and phosphate determination [113,114,117]. In these cases, interference is not caused by the metabolic activity of the cells, but by the glucose conversion with glucose oxidase; this enzyme is coimmobilized with the cells on the transducer surface.

In some cases, we cannot observe any interference in a young biosensor; it gradually appears as the biosensor ages. It can be caused by the activation of other metabolic paths that were repressed during microbe cultivation in a substrate-rich medium—for example, in the lactate biosensor with a yeast *Hansenula anomala* (Table 6.3) [132]. At other times, the growth of a contaminating microbe can be the cause of an increasing degree of interference, for example, in the arginine biosensor with the cells of *Streptococcus faecium* [77]—see also Section 5.2.3.

The whole group of glucose microbial biosensors represents another example of this interference type. Most of them were prepared with the cells that are able to metabolize other sugars as well; the interference degree varies case by case (Table 6.7).

Biosensors with related microbial species can differ according to their response to various interfering substances as we can see, for example, in phenylalanine determination. Two bacterial strains can be used—*Proteus vulgaris* or *P. mirabilis*; in both cases, interference of the same substances is observed, but in different degrees [83].

The bacterial biosensor with *Proteus mirabilis* can use two different potentiometric transducers for the detection of urea hydrolysis: either ammonia or carbon dioxide gas-sensing electrodes. The choice of the transducer type has a significant influence on the spectrum of interfering substances—while in ammonia detection, some amino acids can interfere, the biosensor with a carbon dioxide electrode responds to non-nitrogenous compounds [84,94].

In some biosensors, a wide spectrum of interfering substances can be found, as in the above-mentioned yeast lactate biosensor with the cells of *Hansenula anomala* [133] (see Table 6.3) or in the biosensor for formic acid determination with *Pseudomonas oxaliticus*, which also responds to pyruvate, lactate, acetaldehyde, acetate, and (to a lesser extent) to other organic compounds [73]. On the other hand, there are many cases where we can find only one major interfering substance. In a glutamate biosensor with a squash slice it is pyruvate [34]; in catecholamine determination with the biosensor based on a spinach leaf, a high activity of glycolate oxidase is the source of glycolate interference [130]. The hybrid biosensor for NAD^+ estimation responds to glutamine because of a high glutaminase activity in the cells of *Escherichia coli* [113]. The lactate biosensor with human erythrocytes is specific to this substrate with the exception of malate [7]. The microbial biosensor for methanol determination gives the same response to methanol and ethanol, while the biosensor intended for ethanol determination, based on the cells of another microbial strain, does not respond to methanol at all [51,52].

The presence of other metabolic pathways is not always manifested only by the increase of a measured signal as it was described in all of the examples mentioned up to this time. The capability of microbial cells for metabolizing ammonia is responsible for the signal reduction in those cases in which ammonia is measured as a reaction product [36,37,86].

5.2.3 Influence of Metabolic Pathways of Contaminating Microbes

The cultivation of microbial cells and all handling of them must be kept sterile. If the microbe culture is contaminated by other bacterial cells, their different metabolism can appear as the cause of interference of other substances, as opposed to the case when a pure culture and sterile procedures were used. It is typical that the degree of interference progressively rises as the contaminating bacterial cells, present first in a small amount, grow and multiply.

The following examples can be given: the arginine bacterial biosensor with *Streptococcus faecium* also responds to glutamine and asparagine as a result of bacterial contamination [77]. The biosensor for ammonia determination with nitrifying bacteria is sensitive to glucose, although this bacterial strain is not able to metabolize this sugar. During nitrifying bacteria isolation from activated sludges, all concomitant bacterial strains assimilating glucose were evidently not removed [89].

It is necessary to mention the fact that bacteria isolated from activated sludges and soil are often used for the construction of biosensors applied in measuring the biological oxygen demand in waste water [26,55,58,59]. In this case, it is desirable for the biosensor to respond to the greatest amount of organic compounds possible, and contamination with other microbial strains, as a cause of unselectivity, enables just this use of the biosensor.

CHAPTER 6

Methods of Selectivity Improvement of Cell-Based Biosensors

It can be seen from all foregoing examples that the degree of specificity of cell-based biosensors varies a great deal. Some of them are quite specific; although the selectivity of other biosensors is less, for a given purpose (material type to be analyzed), it can be convenient. The degree of interference not only depends on the character of the interfering substance but also on its concentration in analyzed material. In some cases, interfering substances can make the use of a biosensor for measurements in biological material impossible; such a biosensor is applicable only for the analysis of monocomponental solutions. It is evident that any improvement of the cell-based biosensor selectivity is followed with an enlargement of its practical use. The causes of unselectivity differ, and the degree of interference associated with single compounds varies widely. No wonder so many procedures for selectivity improvement or enhancement exist. They can be based on various principles. Some of them result in a complete interference elimination; the others are only able to improve it to various degrees, which however, can be sufficient for the practical utilization of the biosensor.

In some cases, one procedure is able to enhance the selectivity to an acceptable degree; at other times, it is necessary to combine two, three, or even more methods in order for the biosensor to be useable. The procedure for the selectivity enhancement must be simple enough, accessible, and effective for a long time. The requirement of simplicity is the most important requirement—the cell-based biosensor selectivity may not be enhanced by means of complicated and demanding methods; taken all together, construction of a biosensor with an isolated enzyme could then be more simple and effective.

The following sections classify cell-based biosensors according to the necessity of selectivity improvement and methods used for this purpose; each group is illustrated with numerous concrete examples.

6.1 DETERMINED SUBSTANCE REPRESENTS THE ONLY SOURCE OF CARBON AND/OR ENERGY FOR THE MICROORGANISM

In this case, the substrate is essential for the growth of the microbe species used—no other substrate can be used as a source of carbon or energy. The combination of such microbial cells with a proper transducer results in a biosensor that responds exclusively to this substrate.

This microbe type is used, for example, in a biosensor for methane determination with the cells of *Methylomonas flagellata*. It is a gram-negative, obligate methylotrophic bacterium (i.e., it takes carbon and energy only from methane).

$$CH_4 + NADH + H^+ + O_2 \rightarrow CH_3OH + NAD^+ + H_2O$$

Two methane biosensor types were described. One of them has the microbial cells immobilized in an agar-acetylcellulose membrane on the surface of an oxygen electrode that registers the decrease in oxygen partial pressure [92]. Another possibility is to use a microbial suspension; the analyzed gas comes to the oxygen electrode through this suspension, and a fall in oxygen partial pressure is again registered in comparison with a paired oxygen electrode, to which the same gas is conveyed, passing the cell suspension [22]. Both biosensor types are exclusively selective for methane.

The biosensor proposed for nitrogen dioxide determination with nitrifying bacteria represents another example. Nitrogen dioxide reacts with water and nitrous and nitric acids are formed. Nitrite oxidizing bacteria use nitrite oxidation to nitrate as a sole energy source. The decrease in oxygen concentration is measured with an oxygen electrode, and it is proportional to nitrogen dioxide concentration. This analysis is again highly selective—acetic acid, ethanol, amines, and involatile metabolites (such as glucose or amino acids) do not interfere [93].

Hybrid biosensors for urea or creatinine determination use the substrate transformation in the first reaction catalyzed by isolated enzymes—urease or creatininase. This leads to ammonia production, and this compound is then metabolized in the cells of nitrifying bacteria (*Nitrosomonas sp.* and *Nitrobacter sp.*); the transducer registers the fall in oxygen concentration. Because both of the above-mentioned enzymes are specific for their substrates, and nitrifying bacteria can use only ammonia as an energy source, these hybrid biosensors must be entirely specific [14,15].

6.2 DETERMINED SUBSTANCE IS ESSENTIAL FOR THE GROWTH OF THE MICROBE

Biosensors of this type are, again, from the view of microbe metabolism and growth, wholly specific. Two reactor biosensors for vitamin determination with the cells of the microbial species *Lactobacillus* can serve as examples.

The first of them uses the cells of the microbial strain *Lactobacillus fermenti*, which requires thiamin (vitamin B_1) for its growth. If this vitamin is present in the analyzed solution, the unidentified metabolites are oxidized on a platinum anode that was immersed into the bacterial suspension after its six-hour incubation with the sample; the current increase was proportional to thiamin concentration [23].

Another example is the biosensor for nicotinic acid determination with the cells of *Lactobacillus arabinosus* in polyacrylamide gel. This vitamin is again essential for the microbe growth. The main metabolic product of this microbial strain, lactic acid, is then detected by a glass electrode as causing a decrease in pH value [97].

The inability to synthesize a special metabolite and the resulting growth dependence on the presence of this substance in a culture medium, can also be a typical property of some bacterial strains. Thus, *Salmonella typhimurium* TA100 needs histidine for its growth. The very interesting way of using this bacterial strain for detection of mutagens has been described. The oxygen electrode with these bacterial cells immobilized on its surface is kept in a nutrient medium without histidine. If a chemical mutagen is added into this solution, the genetically defective strain is reverted back to the wild type which can grow without histidine. The growth of the revertants can be examined as a decrease of oxygen partial pressure due to oxygen consumption during the microbe growth [135].

6.3 USE OF GENETICALLY MANIPULATED MICROBIAL STRAINS

These methods use the strains that are deficient in the synthesis of a certain enzyme. The cells can grow if other substrates are present in a culture medium. The folowing examples help to explain how these genetic manipulations can be used to enhance the biosensor selectivity.

Hansenula polymorpha is a yeast that can aerobically metabolize methanol according to the following reaction scheme:

$$CH_3OH \xrightarrow[\text{oxidase}]{\text{alcohol}} HCHO \xrightarrow[\text{dehydrogenase}]{\text{formaldehyde}} HCOOH \xrightarrow[\text{dehydrogenase}]{\text{formate}} CO_2$$

If the yeast strain 34-19 is used on the surface of a pH-sensitive field-effect transistor, a biosensor for methanol determination will be obtained. In contrast to a wild strain, this genetically manipulated yeast is deficient in formate dehydrogenase, and thus a relatively strong formic acid accumulates on the transducer surface and the biosensor sensitivity and its selectivity increase; formic acid cannot interfere with methanol determination as if the wild strain and a carbon dioxide electrode were used [30]. In the yeast strain A3-11, besides the metabolic abnormality described above, another defect of enzyme synthesis appears: the cells cannot metabolize methanol due to the absence of alcohol oxidase. It can be said that the interference of other substrates of the metabolic pathway (methanol and formic acid) shown above was eliminated, and the biosensor that uses these cells is selective for formaldehyde [31].

The yeast cells of *Pichia pinus* can oxidize ethanol with the following intermediates: acetaldehyde−acetic acid−acetyl coenzyme A. The yeast strain 2468 is deficient in acetyl coenzyme A synthetase, and thus it is not able to metabolize acetic acid. The biosensor with these cells is sensitive to ethanol and − in contrast to a biosensor with a wild yeast strain − insensitive to acetic acid [30].

The use of genetically manipulated bacterial strains can be based on the inability of these cells to synthesize a certain substance (vitamin or amino acid), which is then essential for the microbial growth. This strain can be used for the detection of those compounds that are able to revert a deficient strain to a wild type, as it was described at the end of the previous Section 6.2 [135]. *Bacillus subtilis* M45(Rec⁻) was used for the screening of mutagens because it is defective in the DNA recombination enzyme system, as explained in Section 2.3.2 [66].

6.4 MEASURED PRODUCT ORIGINATES EXCLUSIVELY FROM THE ESTIMATED SUBSTRATE

Under given conditions, the measured product cannot originate from substances other than the estimated substrate, therefore the biosensor is, again, entirely specific − e.g., the biosensor for formic acid determination with the cells of *Clostridium buryricum* between two teflon membranes on the surface of a platinum anode. Formic acid is metabolized by the bacterial cells in a four-step reaction; the end-product−gaseous hydrogen−penetrates the teflon membrane, and it is oxidized on the platinum anode. The resulting current is proportional to the formic acid concentration. Metabolization of other volatile compounds (methane, ethanol, acetic acid) cannot be a source of a gaseous hydrogen, and the possible interference of involatile compounds with the transducer is eliminated by another way−see Section 6.5 [136].

The glutamate biosensor is based on the cells of *Escherichia coli* with a high activity of glutamate decarboxylase and a carbon dioxide electrode as a transducer. While under aerobic conditions, this microbe is capable of metabolizing a wide range of substances with carbon dioxide production, under anaerobic conditions any carbon dioxide produced by these bacteria results from the glutamate decarboxylase reaction. The only interfering substance is glutamine, during deamination of which glutamate is produced; its interference, however, can be reduced in another way—see Section 6.7 [33].

Phenylalanine determination is specific if the cell suspension of *Leuconostoc mesenteroides* is used; these cells can produce lactate exclusively from this amino acid. Lactic acid is then estimated with a selective enzyme biosensor based on lactate oxidase and an oxygen electrode [21]. Determination of glucose with a biosensor based on human erythrocytes, which are not able to metabolize other sugars, is specific as well [9].

6.5 ELIMINATION OF THE CONTACT OF INTERFERING SUBSTANCES WITH THE TRANSDUCER

If the interfering substance penetrates as far as the measuring electrode, the electrode responds to its presence, and a false increase in the results ensues. As it was mentioned, this interference type is not only characteristic for cell-based biosensors, but it can be observed in enzyme biosensors as well. Prevention of the diffusion of interfering substances to the transducer can be counted among the possibilities of the biosensor selectivity improvement.

As stated in Section 5.1.3, an ammonium ion-selective membrane electrode is also sensitive to some other cations including Na^+ and K^+ [127]. That is why practically all biosensors based on ammonia detection do not register NH_4^+ ions; instead, they use a gas electrode where a pH-sensitive membrane is covered with a gas-permeable membrane enabling free diffusion of ammonia, but inhibiting the diffusion of any ions. Since the pH-optimum for this electrode operation is about 10.0, which is much higher than the optimal pH of most deaminases and urease, it is necessary to compromise and take a certain fall in sensitivity into account [76,93,123]. Another possibility is to perform the enzyme reaction and the measurement at different pH values. This is also necessary in the case of a conductometric detection of produced ammonia [25].

An anion-exchange membrane can also hinder the diffusion of cations to the ammonium electrode. Neutral and anionic analytes can permeate the positively charged membrane while positively charged interferant species, such as endogenous ammonium and potassium ions, are repelled and, thus, cannot reach the transducer [137].

Many biosensors are based on product detection by its oxidation on an anode. This principle includes, for example, detection of hydrogen peroxide [17,114,119], gaseous hydrogen [55,135] and other reductive substances [23], or a mediator of electron transfer in its reduced form like hexacyanoferrate(II) [2,7,43–46,76] and reduced 2,6-dichlorphenolindophenol [47,128]. In all of these cases, additional substances from analyzed samples can be oxidized on the anode. With respect to their high concentrations in biological fluids, ascorbic and uric acids in particular are the most important interfering substances. The hindrance of their diffusion to the transducer can be reached in several different ways.

Thus, it is possible to remove ascorbic acid from urine samples by means of nonenzymatic oxidation with ferrous chloride and by following treatment of the urine with a katex resin [119] or, enzymatically, with ascorbate oxidase that forms (after immobilization on the biosensor surface) the so-called anti-interference enzyme layer [138].

Electrooxidizable ascorbate and urate can also be completely oxidized by hydrogen peroxide in a peroxidase catalyzed reaction. Peroxidase was immobilized in a layer covering the active electrode, and hydrogen peroxide was either added to the analyzed solution or generated *in situ* by means of a coupled enzyme reaction [140].

Another possibility for the prevention of interference of reducing substances represents the location of an asymmetric acetylcellulose membrane between the cells and the anode [134,140]. The membrane is permeable for hydrogen peroxide, but due to its negative surface charge, it excludes other electrically oxidizable substances that are not electroneutral. Since ascorbic and uric acids are ionized at the working pH of most biosensors, and they are present in solutions as anions, their diffusion to the measuring anode is blocked. This method certainly cannot be used if the measured oxidizable substance is also an anion—for example, hexacyanoferrate(II). Other membranes that exclude the electroactive interferants by size or charge can also be used; they were listed elsewhere [138]. Elimination of the interference of reducing substances in hydrogen peroxide determination on an anode can also be reached by conversion of the measurement to cathodic reduction—see Section 6.16.

Two teflon membranes in the biosensor for formic acid determination, with the cells of *Clostridium butyricum* immobilized between them, also inhibit ionized reducing substances in gaining access to the measuring anode. On the other hand, it enables free diffusion of volatile formic acid to the cells and free diffusion of gaseous hydrogen as a reaction product to the anode [85].

There are several other ways to eliminate the influence of reductive substances on the results—among them are the use of a suitable mode of measurement, or the subtraction of a blank value. These methods will be described in Sections 6.16 and 6.17.

6.6 ELIMINATION OF THE CONTACT OF INTERFERING SUBSTANCES WITH THE CELLS

The interfering substance is metabolized in the cells, and the same product that emerged during the substrate metabolization can emerge now. If we hinder the interferant in its diffusion to the cells, while a free diffusion of the measured substance is not touched, the interfering substance cannot be metabolized, and this arrangement results in a biosensor selectivity improvement.

The easiest way to eliminate contact with the cells is to remove the interfering substance from the analyzed sample. Thus, in sucrose determination with the hybrid biosensor using invertase and microbial cells of *Zymomonas mobilis* rich in glucose-fructose oxidoreductase, glucose and fructose interfere when they are present in the analyzed solution at the same time. That is to say, these sugars are not only products of sucrose splitting, but they are also substrates of the above-mentioned enzyme in the bacterial cells. If glucose oxidase is added into the analyzed sample, glucose is removed, and fructose alone does not interfere with the measurement if an appropriate procedure is applied [112].

Glucose content in the measured solution can modify the result in other hybrid biosensors as well, if it is a product of the first enzyme reaction and, at the same time, a substrate in the second reaction; this remains true even if the enzyme in the cells catalyzes the first [114–116,118] or the second reaction [39]. If hydrogen peroxide is the detected substance, the concept of the so-called enzyme anti-interference layer covering the proper biosensor could be used (Figure 6.1). This anti-interference layer with two coimmobilized enzymes—glucose oxidase and catalase—was used, in the case of a bienzyme biosensor, for α-amylase activity determination, and it enabled the elimination of glucose interference up to its concentration level of 80 mmol/l in biological material [141].

Interference of involatile compounds can be excluded by a gas-permeable membrane that covers the cells. This procedure was used in the biosensor for ethanol detection, with the yeast *Trichosporon brassicae* immobilized in an acetylcellulose membrane on the surface of an oxygen electrode. Since this microbe can metabolize a great number of organic compounds, the cell layer is still covered with a teflon membrane. This membrane prevents diffusion of involatile metabolites, including glucose. If a neutral pH

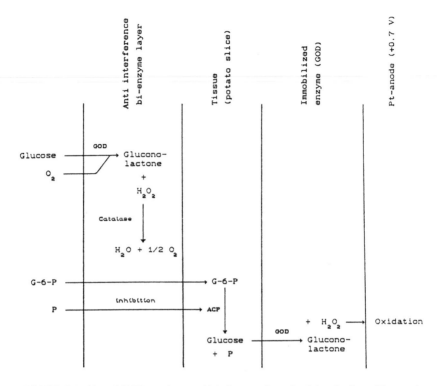

FIGURE 6.1. Use of GOD-catalase anti-interference layer in determination of inorganic phosphate by a hybrid biosensor in glucose containing samples: GOD—glucose oxidase, ACP—acid phosphatase, P—inorganic phosphate, G-6-P—glucose-6-phosphate. (Adapted after Renneberg, R., F. Scheller, K. Riedel, E. Litschko, and M. Richter. 1983. *Anal. Lett.*, 16(B 12):877–890. By courtesy of Marcel Dekker, Inc.)

value of the working solution is used, neither acetic acid nor propionic acid can pass through the membrane because they are fully ionized at this pH. Consequently, only volatile compounds like ethanol, propanol, or butanol can reach the cells [51,52].

The same principle of selectivity enhancement (i.e., the use of a gas-permeable membrane covering the immobilized cells) is used in the biosensor for determination of methanol with the unidentified bacterial strain AJ 3993 on the surface of an oxygen electrode [51,52], or for ethanol estimation with the cells of *Acetobacter aceti* immobilized in calcium alginate gel on the surface of a field-effect transistor sensitive to H⁺ ions [28]. On the contrary, the teflon membrane cannot be used in those cases when the mediator for electron transfer is used in the function of the ethanol cell-based biosensor; hexacyanoferrate(III) must freely diffuse to the cells, which would not be possible through a gas-permeable membrane [43,44].

The teflon membrane covering the cells of *Pseudomonas sp.* on the surface of an oxygen electrode also allows only volatile compounds to reach the cells. The biosensor can be used for carbon dioxide detection; acetic acid only represents an interfering substance — this acid is not ionized at an acidic pH, which is necessary for a free carbon dioxide diffusion and, thus, passes through the membrane and is metabolized in the bacterial cells [138].

Also, an ammonia biosensor with nitrifying bacteria (*Nitrosomonas* and *Nitrobacter sp.*) immobilized in an acetylcellulose membrane on the surface of an oxygen electrode, is covered with a teflon membrane. These microorganisms, isolated from activated sludges, are specific for ammonia, but they are often attended by concomitant bacteria that can assimilate glucose and acetic acid. The teflon membrane does not allow these involatile compounds to get to the cells, and therefore, the metabolism of concomitant microbes cannot become evident [11,52].

6.7 PERMEABILIZATION OF THE CELL MEMBRANE

Intact, vital cells are used for the biosensor construction in most cases. Nevertheless, some authors artificially increase the cell membrane permeability — either with a careful procedure (keeping most of the cells alive) or with such methods that undoubtedly kill the cells, thus, resulting not only in the increase of cell membrane permeability, but even in the destruction of the whole cell.

Among the physical methods of cell membrane permeabilization we can name: lyophilization [33,41,45–47,76,79], ultrasonic treatment [73–77], or the use of extreme pressure [95]. The treatment of the cells with various organic solvents was also used for this purpose — for example, with 40% dimethylsulfoxide [2,44,46], acetone [34], or 10% toluene [99,112]. The cell membrane permeability can be increased by exposing it to buffer containing chelating agents such as EDTA, which removes divalent cations from the cell membrane. This results in the diffusion of pyridine coenzymes and increased diffusion of formate into the bacterial cells, both being necessary for the formate biosensor function [73]. The cells can be killed with the addition of chloramphenicol [78] or die spontaneously due to the lack of nutrients [8].

Lyophilization is the most common procedure of all those mentioned above. The aim of this method is to increase the cell membrane permeability, and to ensure a long-term storability of the cells with a high activity of a special enzyme [41,45].

In general, we can say that if the enzyme is located intracellularly, the increase in cell membrane permeability will facilitate the substrate to get to the enzyme, resulting in a higher sensitivity, and in many cases, in a shorter response time of the biosensor. If the influence of interfering substances remains unaltered (e.g., oxidation of ascorbic and uric acids on the anode), a third result also appears – the biosensor selectivity increases. But in another situation, if the enzyme can be found near the cell surface, and the substrate diffusion through the membrane is quick enough, it is not necessary for the cells to undergo any previous treatment before their use for the biosensor construction. As an example, we can mention ethanol determination with the cells of *Gluconobacter suboxidans*, when the steady state is reached within 30 s (i.e., with the same speed as if the enzyme electrode is used with isolated alcohol dehydrogenase). In this case, any increase of the cell membrane permeability would not improve the biosensor selectivity [43].

Sometimes, the cell membrane is almost impermeable for the substrate, and its permeabilization is necessary for the enhancement of the biosensor sensitivity. The change in the ratio between diffusion speeds of the estimated substrate and potentially interfering substances through the cell membrane must result in the change of the biosensor selectivity. Therefore, in glucose determination with the biosensor using a mould mycelium of *Aspergillus niger* as a biocatalyzer, the diffusion of the substrate and the electron transport mediator into the cells is enabled by treating mycelium with 40% dimethylsulfoxide [2]. Analogically, the freshly prepared biosensor for hydrogen peroxide determination, based on the use of a high catalase activity in human erythrocytes, is only slightly sensitive. The sensitivity rise during the first two weeks of the biosensor operation can be related to a successive spontaneous lysis of erythrocytes [8]. The necessity of using the treated cells of *Pseudomonas oxaliticus* for the formate biosensor construction was already mentioned earlier in this section [73].

In some cases, the permeabilization of the cell membrane can be a determining factor for the biosensor selectivity. The biosensor, using the cells of *Escherichia coli* on the surface of an oxygen electrode, can serve as an example. If intact microbial cells cultivated in a medium with glycerol are used for the biosensor construction, it will respond to D-lactate and succinate. On the other hand, the biosensor with the same cell type broken under an extreme pressure responds most to pyruvate and pyridine coenzymes NADH and NADPH; these compounds cannot pass through the intact cell membrane. Further selectivity improvement of these two biosensors can be reached with the help of inhibitors and the effect of high temperature on the cells [99] – see also Tables 6.4 and 6.5 and Section 6.10.

The last examples will show how diverse the causes of selectivity enhancement of biosensors with permeabilized cells can be. Thus, the biosensor with the cells of *Escherichia coli* on the surface of a carbon dioxide gas-sensing electrode uses glutamate decarboxylating activity for glutamate determination. Since the microbial cells show a high glutaminase activity at the same time, glutamine is a powerful interfering substance; the biosensor response to glutamine represents 108% of its response to glutamate. If we use lyophilized, acetone-treated bacterial cells for the biosensor construction, its response to glutamine decreases to about one-twelfth of its original value, while the response to glutamate remains unchanged. This selectivity enhancement is explained by a hindrance of active glutamine transport across the cell membrane due to its damage during acetone treatment [33].

The biosensor with microbial cells of *Zymomonas mobilis* on the surface of a glass electrode uses, for glucose or fructose determination, two enzymes present in the cells—glucose-fructose oxidoreductase and gluconolactonase (Figure 6.2). If the microbial cells are permeabilized with 10% toluene before being used for the biosensor construction, it is then highly specific for glucose and fructose, and interference by analogous sugars is negligible. This situation can be explained as follows. Permeabilization of the cells causes the leakage of soluble cofactors and high-energy compounds needed for metabolism of other sugars. On the other hand, glucose and fructose conversion by glucose-fructose oxidoreductase is still possible because this enzyme contains an NADP(H) cofactor that is tightly bound to the active site and cannot be lost from the permeabilized cells; activity of this enzyme is not touched [100].

The hybrid biosensor for sucrose determination is prepared analogically. It contains invertase-rich yeast cells of *Saccharomyces cerevisiae* and isolated glucose oxidase, coimmobilized on the surface of an oxygen electrode. The cells are not used in their natural status—they are used after autolysis; while invertase is firmly bound on the inner side of the cell membrane, cytoplasmatic and other intracellular enzymes leave the cells, and

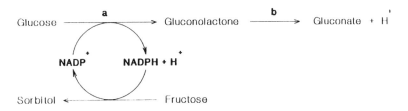

FIGURE 6.2. Principle of glucose or fructose determination by the biosensor with *Zymomonas mobilis* permeabilized cells.

that is why their substrates cannot interfere. The only seriously interfering sugar is glucose; it is the substrate of glucose oxidase that is essential for the biosensor function [142].

6.8 INDUCTION OF ENZYME SYNTHESIS IN MICROBIAL CELLS

Enzymes that are found in the cells of microorganisms (bacteria or yeasts) can be divided into two groups. The first group includes the so-called constitutive enzymes, which are regularly found in the cells and are necessary for a prosperous microbe metabolism. The second group of enzymes are called adaptable or inducible enzymes (i.e., those enzymes whose synthesis is induced only after the cell contact with the enzyme substrate). This means that these enzymes ensure the transformation of less common substrates that the microbes do not encounter regularly. It was demonstrated that inducible enzymes are not present within the cells in the form of an inactive precursor, but there is always the question of enzyme protein synthesis *de novo*—if proteosynthesis is blocked with chloramphenicol, a total repression of the inductor effect on microbial cells can be observed [50].

Enzyme activity in the cell can be increased by induction many times, sometimes even more than ten times, as evidenced from the example in Table 6.1. The effect of this procedure on the biosensor selectivity enhancement is intensified with another result of enzyme synthesis induction. While growth with the substrate results in an increase of a special enzyme

TABLE 6.1. Influence of Twelve-Hour Incubation with Inductor (2 mmol/l) on the Response of Bacillus subtilis *Cell-Based Biosensor to Various Sugars.*

	Increase of the Biosensor Response in % after Preincubation with		
	Sucrose	Maltose	Lactose
Sucrose	2322	83	168
Maltose	83	1905	147
Lactose	—	—	2680
Glucose	96	118	117
Glycerol	82	130	200

Adapted after Riedel, K., R. Renneberg, and F. Scheller. 1990. *Anal. Lett.*, 23(5):757–770. By courtesy of Marcel Dekker, Inc.

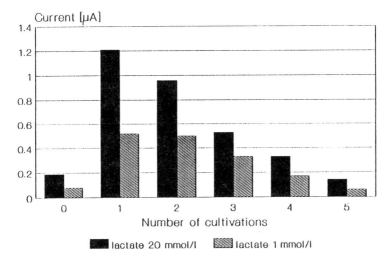

FIGURE 6.3. Changes of lactate dehydrogenase activity of flavocytochrome b_2 in the yeast cells of *Hansenula anomala* during repeated cultivations, expressed as a yeast biosensor response to L-lactate: 0—yeast cells cultivated on a Sabouraudes's agar 1–5—number of cultivations in a liquid medium with L-lactate. (Reprinted from Racek, J. and J. Musil. 1987. *Clin. Chim. Acta,* 162(2):129–139. With permission.)

activity in the cells, at the same time, it can cause a depression in synthesis, and thus, the activity decrease of other intracellular enzymes that would be necessary for the transformation of the substrates which are just absent in the culture medium [46].

Synthesis induction during microbe cultivation with a substrate was described in the case of enzymes metabolizing sugars, amino acids, and other organic compounds or even inorganic ions; many examples are summarized in Table 6.2.

The complexity of the problems of enzyme induction can be illustrated in the following results. Above all, it is necessary to know that the inductive effect in most cases appears gradually, and in repeated cultivations, enzyme activity can still rise. This knowledge, however, cannot be applied to all cases, and sometimes we observed that, in successive cycles of microbial growth, the enzyme activity within the cells decreased once again – in some cases, considerably. This is the case with the cultivation of *Hansenula anomala* cells in the liquid medium with lactate, which induces synthesis of flavocytochrome b_2 with lactate dehydrogenase activity [45] (Figure 6.3) or with the induction of tyrosine-phenol lyase in the cells of *Aeromonas phenologenes* by tyrosine [80]. The authors tried to explain this observation by the long-term development of alternative metabolic degradation path-

TABLE 6.2. Examples of Biosensors Based on Microbial Cells
Prepared during Incubation in Liquid Medium with the Inductor.

Microbe Type	Inductor	Reference
Aeromonas phenologenes	Tyrosine	[81]
Arthrobacter nicotiana	Butyric acid	[129]
Aspergillus niger	Glucose	[2]
Azotobacter vinelandii	Potassium nitrate	[36]
Bacillus subtilis	Glucose	[39,50,57]
	Maltose	[39]
	Glutamate*	[57,144]
	Aspartame	[147]
	Peptides	[40]
Chemiautotrophic thermo- philic bacteria	KHCO$_3$	[158]
Enterobacter agglomerans	Ascorbic acid	[6]
Escherichia coli	Glutamate	[33]
	Tryptophane	[91]

	D,L-Lactate,
	  glycerol, suc-
	  cinate, D,L-
	  malate
		[99]

Hansenula anomala	Glucose	[101]
	Lactate*	[45–47, [121,151]
Hyphomicrobium sp.	Methylsulfate*	[79]
Nocardia erythropolis	Cholesterol	[78]
Nocardia opaca	Androstendione	[128]
Pseudomonas fluorescens	Glucose	[48,159]
	Tryptophane	[96]
Pseudomonas oxalaticus	Formic acid	[73]
Pseudomonas sp.	Histidine	[37]
	Nitrilotriacetic acid	[86]
	KHCO$_3$	[143]
	Proline*	[145]
Saccharomyces cerevisiae	Glucose	[49]
Serratia marcescens	Asparagine	[95]
Streptococcus mutans	Glucose	[20]
Thiobacillus ferrooxidans	Fe^{2+}	[102]
Thiobacillus thioparus	Thiosulfate	[122]
Trichosporon cutaneum	Phenol	[41]
Zymomonas mobilis	Glucose	[100,112]

*Inductor represents the only source of carbon and energy during the microbe cultivation.

48

ways for the substrate. That is why they recommend keeping microbes on common culture media and, only before the biosensor construction, to inoculate the cells into a substrate-rich solution. Another possibility is to store induced cells after their lyophilization [45].

The highest induction degree can be obtained in the case when the microbial cells are cultivated in a medium with the substrate as a sole source of carbon and energy for the cell growth [45,46,79,143–145]. A total repression of synthesis of other enzymes is not unusual in these cases, which results in a high biosensor selectivity for the substrate. Thus, in the cultivation of the yeast *Hansenula anomala*, L-lactate can represent the only carbon source, and this substrate causes a very high degree of induction of lactate-converting flavocytochrome b$_2$ synthesis [146]. The yeast cells prepared in this way and placed on the surface of a platinum anode form the highly selective biosensor for lactate determination. When the biosensor was freshly prepared, none of the thirty-one substances tested – including amino acids, glucose, pyruvate, ketone bodies, and ethanol – interfered with the lactate determination. This exclusive selectivity lasts for one week; as the biosensor ages, we can observe an increasing interference of some organic compounds, and after one month the biosensor selectivity is quite poor [135] (Table 6.3). This is caused by a gradual activation of synthesis of other enzymes during the biosensor operation.

Some researchers solve this problem by keeping the biosensor with living microbial cells in a medium containing the measured substrate [36,91,95]. Sometimes the biosensor can gain its selectivity only during repeated measurements, as in the case of the biosensor for sulfite determination with the cells of *Thiobacillus thioparus* on an oxygen electrode. The growth of this chemoautotrophic aerobic bacterium could not be observed in the medium containing sodium sulfite as a sulfur source; for this reason, the bacterial cells are grown in a thiosulfate-containing medium. If these cells are used for the biosensor preparation, its response to thiosulfate is much higher than its response to sulfite. In order to condition the immobilized bacterial cells to the sulfite ion, the biosensor was used only for the measurement of sulfite. As a result, the response to sulfite increased day-by-day whereas the response to thiosulfate decreased gradually (Figure 6.4). After four days, the biosensor response to sulfite became stable, and it was almost eight times higher than its response to thiosulfate [122].

Various substrates can induce synthesis of different enzymes in the cells of one microbial species. These cells can be used for the construction of several biosensors that differ in their substrate specificity. Thus, induced bacterial cells of *Bacillus subtilis*, immobilized on the surface of an oxygen electrode, are a basis of biosensors for the estimation of glucose [68], glutamate [144], aspartame [147], various peptides and proteases [40], sugars,

TABLE 6.3. Interference of Some Metabolites and Drugs with Lactate Determination by a Yeast Biosensor with Hansenula anomala *and Its Changes during the Biosensor Aging.*

	Biosensor Response (Response to Lactate = 100%)				
	0	7	15	21	30 d
Lactate:	100.0	100.0	100.0	100.0	100.0
Pyruvate	0	0	3.3	10.5	25.8
Serine	0	0	2.1	9.4	24.4
Glycine	0	0	1.7	7.2	19.2
Alanine	0	0	1.7	6.3	19.2
Glutamate	0	0	5.1	14.7	15.7
Aspartate	0	0	3.1	4.2	15.7
Glycerol	0	0	0.5	1.1	9.1
Lysine	0	0	0.1	1.0	9.1
Glucose	0	0	0.8	1.6	7.7
Leucine	0	0	0.2	1.0	7.7
Citrulline	0	0	0.2	1.2	7.3
Histidine	0	0	0.5	0.7	7.3
Ethanol	0	0	0.5	0.8	7.0
Arginine	0	0	0.1	0.4	6.4
Isoleucine	0	0	0.1	0.9	6.3
Glutamine	0	0	0.2	0.6	5.6
Sorbitol	0	0	0.2	0.5	5.2
Phenylalanine	0	0	0.3	0.6	4.9
Galactose	0	0	0	0.9	4.2
3-Hydroxybutyrate	0	0	0.2	1.1	4.1
Ethylene glycol	0	0	0	1.0	4.0
Valine	0	0	0.3	0.8	3.5
Acetoacetate	0	0	0	1.1	3.3
Fructose	0	0	0	1.3	3.1
2-Oxoglutarate	0	0	0	1.1	2.8
Mannitol	0	0	0	0.3	2.1
Malate	0	0	0	0	2.1
Salicylate	0	0	0	0	1.7
Acetone	0	0	0	0	0

Reprinted from Racek, J. and J. Musil. 1987. *Clin. Chim. Acta,* 167(1):59–65. With permission.

amino acids, and glycerol [50], α-amylase [39], or biological oxygen demand [57]. The synthesis of different enzymes can also be induced in the cells of other microbial species as shown in Table 6.2.

The inducing substrate is, in most cases, the cause of the synthesis of such enzyme molecules, which are necessary for its metabolization. But sometimes, other intracellular enzymes can also be induced; the cells prepared in this way can be used for the construction of the biosensor, which is sensitive to a metabolite other than the inductor. As an example, we can show the induction of various flavoprotein oxidases in the cells of *Escherichia coli* — the results are summarized in Table 6.4. This table shows that induced bacterial cells can hardly be used for the construction of the biosensor, which would be selective enough — the cells also metabolize other substrates, although to a lesser extent [99]. An analogic opinion is also found among the authors of other cell-based biosensors that contain the cells cultivated with the inductor. Consequently, it is necessary to use other methods for the selectivity enhancement; among them, inhibition of other metabolic paths is foremost — see also Section 6.10.

The unusual type of enzyme synthesis induction in the cells of *Escherichia coli* was used for the preparation of a hybrid lactose biosensor. The genetically manipulated *E. coli* K-12 recombinant PQ-37 is characterized by the following property: the DNA damage by mutagenic compounds is manifested by increasing the production of the enzyme β-galactosidase; activity of this enzyme in the cells is thirty-fold higher after induction than before it [116].

Induction of enzyme synthesis can be used only in the culture of microorganisms. In biosensors based on immobilization of animal or plant cells, it is necessary to choose the tissue that has the least possible amount of other

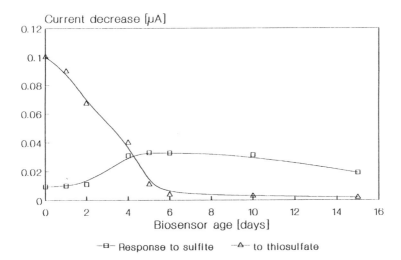

FIGURE 6.4. Substrate specificity change of the biosensor with *Thiobacillus thioparus* cells during measurements of sulfite containing samples. (Reprinted from Suzuki, M., S. Lee, K. Fujii, I. Arikawa, I. Kubo, T. Kanagawa, E. Mikami, and I. Karube. 1992. *Anal. Lett.,* 25(6):973–982. By courtesy of Marcel Dekker, Inc.)

TABLE 6.4. *Influence of Growth in a Medium with Various Inductors (10 g/l) on the Respiratory Activity of the Cells Escherichia coli in the Presence of Given Substrates (50 mmol/l).*

Inductor	Bacterial Cells	Respiratory Activity in μmol O_2/min·mg of Proteins						
		NADH	NADPH	D-Lactate	L-Lactate	Succinate	L-Malate	Pyruvate
Glycerol	Whole	0.3	<0.1	1.5	0.3	1.5	0	0
	Broken	6.0	1.5	1.5	0.3	2.2	0	15.0
D,L-Lactate	Whole	0.4	<0.1	1.5	30.0	3.0	0	0
Succinate	Whole	0.4	<0.1	0.7	3.7	3.7	0	0
D,L-Malate	Whole	0.1	<0.1	6.0	5.4	5.4	6.7	0

Reprinted from Burstein, C., E. Adamowicz, K. Boucherit, C. Rabouille, and J.-L. Romette. 1986. *Appl. Biochem. Biotechnol.*, 12(1):1-16. With permission.

metabolic paths. Nevertheless, in these cases too, we often cannot manage without the use of other ways of selectivity enhancement, such as inhibition of other enzymes, choice of a suitable working pH, etc. In spite of it, the possibility of enzyme induction is not quite excluded even here. Thus, rat liver microsomes were used for the sulfite biosensor construction after the animals had been treated with phenobarbital and 5,6-benzoflavone [148]. Similarly, liver microsomes from rats treated with ascorbic acid were utilized to measure ascorbate with the organelle electrode [148]. This treatment leads to an increase of enzyme synthesis in liver cells of experimental animals.

6.9 CHOICE OF pH SUITABLE FOR THE ANALYSIS

A suitable pH value of the working solution can improve the biosensor selectivity on the basis of two different principles. Ionization of organic or inorganic interfering compounds can appear due to a change in pH value; then, the ionized compound cannot pass through a gas-permeable membrane. The second principle is based on a different pH-optima in the substrate-converting enzyme and the other enzyme, which catalyzes such a reaction of interfering substance, in which the same product originates. Also, the latter principle is based on a different ionization of functional groups, this time in the active center of enzyme molecules. We can show two examples of the principles metioned above.

As shown in Section 6.6, the biosensor with the cells of *Trichosporon brassicae* on the surface of an oxygen electrode responds only to volatile compounds (alcohols) if the cells are covered with a teflon membrane and the operational pH equals 7.0 [51,52]. If the biosensor arrangement remains unchanged, but the working pH falls to 3.0, the same biosensor also starts to respond to acetic, propionic, and butyric acids. At this pH value the ionization of these weak organic acids is suppressed, and they are suddenly able to pass across the teflon membrane – thus, they can be metabolized by the yeast cells [52,53].

The cysteine bacterial biosensor is based on the cell suspension of *Proteus morganii* on the surface of a membrane gas electrode sensitive to hydrogen sulfide. The transducer responds not only to this product, but also to carbon dioxide produced in the cells during urea hydrolysis; urea thus represents a significant interfering substance. At a pH of 5.0, the biosensor response to carbon dioxide is 1.93 times higher than the biosensor response to hydrogen sulfide. Since the pK_a value of hydrogen sulfide (7.0) is greater than that of carbon dioxide (6.7), some improvement in selectivity for H_2S would be expected by working at higher pH values. Indeed, at a pH value of

7.45, the biosensor response to cysteine is 1.7 times higher than that to urea. However, this selectivity improvement is not sufficient enough for the biosensor to be used in practice [85].

Two tissue electrodes can serve as examples of enzyme activity suppression at an appropriate pH value. The first example uses a slice of a porcine kidney on the surface of an ammonia gas electrode for glucosamine-6-phosphate detection. The transducer registers ammonia – the product of the substrate deamination. Glutaminase, which is also present in the kidney tissue, is the cause of glutamine interference. Fortunately, there is a lot of difference in the pH-optima for glucosamine-6-phosphate and glutamine deamination, and moreover, the relative biocatalytic activity of porcine kidney tissue for glucosamine-6-phosphate is substantially higher than that for glutamine. That is why this tissue biosensor is, with a pH of 9.25, sufficiently selective for glucosamine-6-phosphate [110] (Figure 6.5).

The biosensor for adenosine determination uses mucosal cells from the small intestine of a mouse that have a high activity of adenosine deaminase; the deamination product – ammonia – is measured with a gas electrode. Adenine-containing nucleotides (AMP, ADP, and ATP) can interfere because they can be deaminated with nucleotide deaminases. Nevertheless, if we choose pH 9.0 for the working buffer, it represents the pH-optimum for adenosine deaminase, whereas the pH-optima for nucleotide

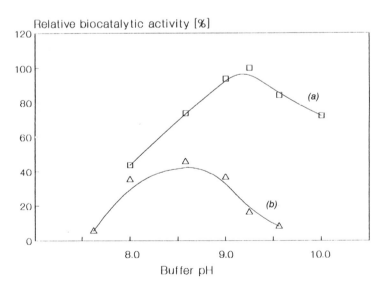

FIGURE 6.5. Comparison of pH profiles for glucosamine-6-phosphate (a) and glutamine (b) with the porcine kidney tissue-based biosensors. (Reprinted from Ma, Y. L. and G. A. Rechnitz. 1985. *Anal. Lett.*, 18(B 13):1635–1646. By courtesy of Marcel Dekker, Inc.)

deaminases are substantially lower. These enzymes are, at a pH value of 9.0, practically inactive [32].

6.10 INHIBITION OF ENZYMES OF OTHER METABOLIC PATHWAYS

Interference due to the presence of other metabolic pathways belongs to the most important types in cell-based biosensors and often limits their practical use. This interference type can be observed in microorganisms and tissues of higher plants or animals. Therefore, it is best to choose those microbial strains whose metabolism is intended for the transformation of a determined substance. It can either be an obligatory property of the cells, or it is achieved during microbe cultivation with the substrate. In contrast to microorganisms, whose cells must perform all metabolic functions, the tissues are often so extremely specialized that activity of a special enzyme is very high, while some other metabolic pathways can even be absent, such as in mammalian erythrocytes. In spite of this, enzymes of other metabolic pathways can also cause the interference in tissue biosensors, and it is then necessary to search for inhibitors that would suppress their effect.

Glucose is, among interfering substances, the most common—it can be metabolized by most microorganisms and tissues. Several procedures for the hindrance of glucose interference have been proposed; all of them are based on the addition of glycolyse inhibitors to the analyzed sample, if reversible inhibition is in question, or on the treatment of microbial cells with irreversible glycolyse inhibitors. In the case of the lactate biosensor with the cells of *Hansenula anomala,* glucose interference was completely suppressed by adding sodium fluoride to a working buffer [132]. The same method was used in a biosensor with *Bacillus subtilis*, intended for glutamate determination. Another method—irreversible inhibition of glycolysis in bacterial cells by chlormercuribenzoate—was also applied in this case [143]. Glycolysis in a slice of a porcine kidney used in glutamine determination was successfully suppressed by iodacetamide [13]. This inhibitor was also used in the pyruvate biosensor based on carbon dioxide production in the cells of *Streptococcus faecium*. In this case it was necessary, besides glycolysis inhibition, to suppress the influence of tyrosine; in its decarboxylation in bacterial cells carbon dioxide is produced as well. It was found that adding tyramine reduces tyrosine interference to about one-third [82].

Special enzyme inhibitors can also improve the selectivity of the tyrosine biosensor, which is based on the cells of *Aeromonas phenologenes*, on the surface of an ammonia electrode. Glutamine interference was eliminated by a repeated dialysis in a solution of 6-diazo-5-oxo-L-norleucine, which is known to be an irreversible competitive inhibitor of glutaminase. The influence of glycine, serine, and threonine was suppressed with a dialysis in iodacetamide solution. In spite of all of these procedures, the biosensor selectivity was not sufficient, and some other amino acids (especially asparagine) interfered with tyrosine determination [80]. Authors of the hybrid biosensor for NAD$^+$ determination, which contains *Escherichia coli* cells and an ammonia electrode, mentioned the possibility of glutaminase inhibition by iodacetate or by glutamate, which is the product of a glutaminase catalyzed reaction [113].

Many biosensors are based on the detection of ammonia by a special electrode. Since many microbes can assimilate ammonia and, thus, reduce the measured values, adding isonicotinic acid hydrazide to the analyzed solution is recommended. This compound, in concentrations between 0.1 and 1.0 mmol/l, is known to be an effective competitive inhibitor of aminotransferases, which are involved in ammonia assimilation. This method was used in biosensors for the detection of nitrilotriacetic acid [85] and histidine [37] with the cells of *Pseudomonas sp.* and in nitrate determination with *Azotobacter vinelandii* [36].

The tissue adenosine biosensor with mucosal cells from the small intestine of a mouse is also not very selective. Adenosine-containing nucleotides can interfere in two different ways. The first way – direct deamination – is common for all nucleotides; the second concerns adenosine monophosphate only – it can be hydrolyzed to adenosine with alkaline phosphatase from the intestine mucosal cells. Direct deamination can be suppressed at an appropriate pH value of the working solution (see Section 6.9); intestinal alkaline phosphatase is selectively inhibited by L-phenylalanine [31].

The tissue guanine biosensor uses guanine transformation to xanthine and ammonia in a rat liver tissue on the surface of an ammonia gas electrode. Guanosine can interfere because it is converted to guanine in a guanosine phosphorylase catalyzed reaction. Since this enzyme needs inorganic phosphate as a cosubstrate, phosphate removal from the buffer system results in the elimination of guanosine interference. Adenosine-containing nucleotides represent another group of interfering substances. They can be converted to adenosine due to high alkaline phosphatase activity in liver tissue; adenosine then liberates ammonia under the influence of hepatic adenosine deaminase. This interference can be eliminated by Mn^{2+} ions, which in a concentration of 10 mmol/l, completely inhibit adenosine deaminase activity [103].

And finally, here is one more example when the use of proper inhibitors is an important part of a complex approach to biosensor selectivity improvement. The cells of *Escherichia coli*, in connection with an oxygen

TABLE 6.5. *Preparation of Substrate-Specific Microbial Biosensors with the Cells* Escherichia coli *by Means of Enzyme Induction, Permeabilization of the Cell Membrane, Addition of Inhibitors, and Treatment with a High Temperature.*

Substrate	Inductor	Permeability for Substrate	Inhibitor of Substrate Assimilation	Thermo-sensitivity
3-Phospho-glycerol	Glycerol	Yes	–	Yes
Succinate	Succinate	Yes	Fumarate, Malonate	No
L-Lactate	D,L-Lactate	Yes	Pyruvate	Yes
D-Lactate	*	Yes	Pyruvate	Yes
L-Malate	D,L-Malate	Yes	Oxaloacetate	Yes
Pyruvate	*	No	–	No
NAD(P)H	*	No	–	Yes

*Metabolized with a constitutive enzyme. Reprinted from Burstein, C., E. Adamowicz, K. Boucherit, C. Rabouille, and J.−L. Romette. 1986. *Appl. Biochem. Biotechnol.,* 12(1):1–16. With permission.

electrode, can form biosensors intended for the analysis of D-lactate, L-lactate, L-malate, 3-glycerol phosphate, pyruvate, succinate, or NAD(P)H. The first precondition for obtaining the cells suitable for the analysis of a special substance is the induction of enzyme synthesis during cultivation in a medium with the substrate to be determined, which was already shown in Section 6.8. As the biosensors prepared with these cells would not be selective enough (see Table 6.4), it is necessary to complete enzyme induction with other methods for selectivity improvement, namely with cell membrane permeabilization (see Section 6.7), and, above all, with the use of special inhibitors for alternative metabolic pathways. The results of these procedures are summarized in Table 6.5; microbial biosensors with a very good selectivity to single substrates can be obtained [99].

6.11 PREVENTION OF TRANSPORT OF INTERFERING SUBSTANCE ACROSS THE CELL MEMBRANE

If we succeed in finding the way to hinder the diffusion of interfering substance into the cell while the free transport of a determined substrate is unchanged, we can again observe the biosensor selectivity enhancement.

Thus, in the tyrosine biosensor with the cells of *Aeromonas phenolo-*

genes, besides a glutaminase inhibitor [80], a γ-L-glutamylhydrazide addition can also be used for the elimination of glutamine interference. This compound blocks the glutamine transport across the bacterial membrane. It is especially to use a combination of the procedures mentioned above; that is, glutaminase inhibition and a glutamine transport block result in a marked fall in the biosensor response to glutamine, the interference of which becomes negligible [150].

The hindrance of glutamine transport into bacterial cells, this time into *Escherichia coli* cells, can also be achieved with acetone treatment of the cell membrane as mentioned in Section 6.7, dealing with the cell membrane permeabilization [33].

In fact, the effect of chlormercuribenzoate on the cells of *Bacillus subtilis*, eliminating glucose interference in glutamate determination, is explained by the hindrance of glucose receipt by the bacterial cells [144].

6.12 ACTIVATION OF THE SUBSTRATE-CONVERTING ENZYME

If the activity of a substrate-converting enzyme in the cells increases and activity of other intracellular enzymes remains unchanged, it results in an improvement of the cell-based biosensor selectivity. This can be achieved by enzyme synthesis induction during microbe cultivation with the substrate (see Section 6.8), or with the addition of suitable enzyme activators.

Thus, in the serine-sensitive biosensor with the cells of *Clostridium acidiurici*, the addition of iron(II) stearate to the bacterial paste activates serine dehydratase and the use of dithiothreitol in the working solution protects sulfhydryl groups of this enzyme from oxidation [80]. Dithiothreitol used in washing solutions also protects formate dehydrogenase in the cells of *Pseudomonas oxalaticus* in formic acid determination [73] and L-aspartase in the cells of *Bacterium cadaveris*, in aspartate determination [87].

Lactase in the cells of *Escherichia coli*, which are used for the lactose hybrid biosensor construction, increases its activity by two times after the addition of Mn^{2+} ions and β-mercaptoethanol [116]. Bacterial glutaminase is significantly activated by Mn^{2+} ions; that is why manganese chloride is contained in the working solution of the glutamine-sensitive biosensor with the cells of *Sarcina flava* [13,88].

6.13 PREVENTION OF GROWTH OF CONTAMINATING MICROBES

The bacterial biosensor using cell suspension of *Streptococcus lactis* measures ammonia produced in the first and fourth reaction of a multi-step arginine degradation, and it is highly selective for this amino acid — no response was found in seventeen different amino acids and urea [120]. It was, thus, a surprise that the biosensor with related cells of *Streptococcus faecium*, the metabolism of which is similar, responds to arginine as well as to glutamine and asparagine, and partially to other amino acids and urea [77]. During the following study, glutamine and asparagine interference was found to be a function of the age of the electrode. On the first day there was very little response to glutamine, but it steadily increased and by the seventh day it was practically the same as the response to arginine. It was confirmed that the interference was caused by contaminating gram-negative bacteria that are able to metabolize asparagine and glutamine. An effective preventive procedure was proposed: between the measurements, the biosensor was stored in a buffer containing sodium azide in a concentration of 1.0 mmol/l. It is known that azide inhibits the growth of aerobic bacteria by binding to the iron of the cytochrome porphyrin ring, thus, preventing their oxido-reductive function. On the contrary, *Streptococcus faecium*, like other lactic-acid bacteria, lacks a cytochrome system, and it is therefore unaffected by azide. Using this procedure, the interference of amino acids, including glutamine and asparagine, decreased under 2% of the biosensor response to arginine [74].

Similar circumstances can be observed in the case of the ammonia biosensor, which registers ammonia oxidation by nitrifying bacteria from activated sludges. The biosensor response to glucose and other metabolites is very small, but with the biosensor aging, it rises, although nitrifying bacteria themselves do not assimilate them [88]. Essential selectivity improvement appears only after covering the cell layer with a teflon membrane that makes a barrier against the diffusion of involatile compounds to the cells. Their metabolization by contaminating bacterial cells is excluded, while ammonia at a working pH of 10.0 can freely penetrate the teflon membrane [11]. Another possibility for eliminating the growth of contaminating microbes is to add chloramphenicol to the working buffer [89].

6.14 CHOOSING THE OPTIMAL TYPE OF TRANSDUCER

The biosensor selectivity is defined, above all, by the quality of the receptor (i.e., in this case, of microbial cells or the tissue). Despite this fact, the transducer can also be important in biosensor selectivity for a special substrate.

The thermistor thermometer represents the least selective transducer. The cell-based thermistor with the yeast *Saccharomyces cerevisiae*, immobilized in polyacrylamide gel, registers assimilation of any substrate during its passage through the column with the cells due to temperature increase [27].

The oxygen electrode is the most common transudcer type met in the construction of cell-based biosensors. Several cases can be found where an oxygen electrode also participates in the biosensor selectivity, but they are very rare (see next paragraph). More often it is used for the registration of microbe respiration, that is, vital processes during which oxygen is consumed, no matter which substrate is metabolized. This principle is used, for example, for biological oxygen demand estimation as a criterion of water pollution with organic substances, or in the determination of antimicrobial or antitumor drugs, which will be discussed in greater detail in Section 6.19.

Now, we will see examples where the type of transducer used is a determining factor for the biosensor specificity. The biosensors of this group use the same tissue or microbe species, and the transducer determines the substrate that will cause the biosensor response.

Yellow squash or cucumber fructus contains ascorbate oxidase and glutamate decarboxylase in high activities. By combining this tissue with the oxygen electrode, we obtain the biosensor for ascorbic acid determination [6,42]. On the other hand, if the same tissue slice is placed on the surface of a carbon dioxide electrode, the biosensor responds to glutamate [34]. The selectivity of both biosensor types is so high that it is not necessary to improve it by any other way.

Human erythrocytes are highly specialized cells having only a limited amount of active metabolic paths. No wonder that, in combination with a proper transducer, we obtain a selective biosensor. Thus, erythrocyte suspension on the surface of an oxygen electrode can be used as a specific biosensor for hydrogen peroxide estimation because of the high catalase activity in these cells [8]. The same suspension held on the surface of a glass electrode registers a decrease in pH value during glucose assimilation in the cells [9]. Lastly, if we place human erythrocytes on the platinum anode and add coenzyme NAD^+ with potassium hexacyanoferrate(III) and phenazine methosulfate as electron transfer mediators, the high lactate dehydrogenase activity in the cells is manifested, and the biosensor selectively responds with the current increase to lactate [7]. A survey of erythrocyte-based biosensors is shown in Table 6.6.

The biosensor with *Escherichia coli* cells and a carbon dioxide electrode uses glutamate decarboxylase activity for glutamate determination [33]. Tryptophanase activity in the cells of the same bacterial strain is manifested if they are combined with an ammonia gas-sensing electrode, and tryptophane concentration can thus be measured [90]. Finally, the cells of *Escherichia coli* on the surface of an oxygen electrode constitute the biosensor that uses oxidation of corresponding substrates for determination of D- and L-lactate, L-malate, succinate, pyruvate, glycerol phosphate, or NAD(P)H

TABLE 6.6. Examples of Various Erythrocyte-Based Biosensors in Dependence on the Type of a Transducer.

Substrate	Transducer	Active Enzyme	Product	Ref.
Lactate	Platinum anode	Lactate dehydrogenase (E.C. 1.1.1.27)	$Fe(CN)_6^{4-}$	[7]
Hydrogen peroxide	Oxygen electrode	Catalase (E.C. 1.11.1.6)	O_2	[8]
Glucose	Glass electrode	Enzymes of a glycolytic pathway	H^+	[9]

[99]. It is necessary to point out that all of the biosensors with the cells of *Escherichia coli* mentioned above are prepared with the substrate induced cells; besides a proper transducer type, enzyme induction is also responsible for the biosensor selectivity.

In all of the examples given so far, the biosensors had the same receptor, that is, the same microbe or tissue type; only the transducer decided which metabolic pathway would be used in the biosensor operation and, thus, which substrate would be determined. Another possibility still exists. Two biosensors can have the same cell type and different transducers, but both transducers will examine the same metabolic process. It is possible if, during the substrate transformation, two different substances are produced (or consumed) for which two different selective transducers exist. Also in this arrangement, a different selectivity can be observed if the interfering metabolic pathway is the source of only one of the measured products or if the interfering substance influences only one transducer type.

The biosensor for urea determination with the cells of *Proteus mirabilis* can be ranked with this biosensor group. Urea hydrolysis by urease in the cells can be registered as ammonia or carbon dioxide production with special potentiometric gas sensors. Influence of other metabolic pathways, and thus interference of various substances, differ in both cases as discussed in greater detail in Section 5.2.2 [84].

In oxalate determination with the biosensor containing an acetone-treated banana skin, oxalate oxidase is responsible for the biosensor function; it splits oxalate into two molecules of carbon dioxide and one molecule of hydrogen peroxide. Both of these compounds can be examined electrochemically—if a carbon dioxide gas-sensing electrode is used, reducing substances (like ascorbic acid) cannot interfere, but the biosensor sensitivity is by one order lower than if hydrogen peroxide production is measured by its oxidation on the anode [115].

Lactate oxidation in the yeast cells of *Hansenula anomala* can be examined as a decrease in oxygen partial pressure with a Clark electrode, or [after hexacyanoferrate(III) is added] reoxidation of the hexacyanoferrate(II) produced is measured amperometrically. Ascorbic and uric acids can be directly oxidized on the platinum anode and thus interfere with amperometric detection of hexacyanoferrate(II) [46,132]. This interference is excluded if an oxygen electrode is used as a transducer, but in this case, interference of pyruvate and glucose is more pronounced [118].

Transducer selectivity is also very important in the detection of an atypical ion that cannot be found in nature and must be artificially loaded into the cells before their use for the biosensor construction. The use of these cells for the determination of lysozyme [71] and nystatin [70] was described in Section 2.3.3.

6.15 CHOOSING THE OPTIMAL TYPE OF CELLS

Many cases exist where the biosensor for determining a special compound can be prepared with two, three, or even more different cell types. These cells are either microbial, or arranged in tissues, or one of the cell types is combined with an isolated enzyme to form a hybrid biosensor. It is no surprise that different cells and tissues can show a different specificity, yet metabolize the identical substrate. These differences are caused mainly by a different enzyme content in the cells, but other factors can also be held responsible. We can name, for example, the unequal diffusion rate of interfering substances across cell membranes. It is also important that the individual cell types can be combined with different transducers that influence the biosensor selectivity.

The selectivity of all biosensor types for the determination of a special substrate is sometimes exclusive in every case, at other times it is poor. Usually we can find one biosensor type that is more selective and, thus, more convenient for practical use than the others. Nevertheless, the choice of the biosensor that would be best for determining a special substrate depends also on taking other biosensor properties into consideration, such as simplicity and the speed of the biosensor construction, its stability, the response time, and, not lastly, the purpose of the biosensor use. The following paragraphs show several groups of biosensors, all applicable for an identical type of analysis, but with different immobilized cells. The biosensor selectivity for the analyzed substrate is the criterion for their evaluation.

Both cell-based biosensors for hydrogen peroxide determination, using catalase activity of a bovine liver tissue [111] or of human erythrocytes [8], show practically the same selectivity, and other properties are also similar. The same can be said about glutamate biosensors. Three types have been described: two microbial biosensors with the cells of *Escherichia coli* [33] or *Bacillus subtilis* [143] and one tissue biosensor with a slice of a squash fructus [34]. Without any interventions, the tissue biosensor shows the best selectivity, but if we use permeabilized *Escherichia coli* cells or inhibitors of glycolysis in the biosensor with *Bacillus subtilis*, we obtain glutamate biosensors with comparable and, at the same time, very good selectivity. Additionally, both biosensors for nystatin determination with *Saccharomyces cerevisiae* show a good selectivity for this antimycotic drug, although they are based on different principles. One of them registers the decrease in respiratory activity of the cells used [64,65], while the other measures intracellular ions, liberated from the yeasts as a result of the drug action on the cells [70].

Two types of formate-sensitive biosensors are based on degradation of formic acid in the cells of *Clostridium butyricum* or *Pseudomonas oxalaticus*. While the biosensor with the former microbe species is wholly specific [136], the biosensor with the latter cells also responds to pyruvate, lactate, acetaldehyde, and to a lesser extent to some other metabolites [73]. Also, in ascorbic acid determination, the tissue electrode is more selective than the microbial biosensor with the cells of *Enterobacter agglomerans*. In the tissue biosensor, only isoascorbic acid interferes, and glucose and fructose give a response that is equal to 7.5% of that to ascorbic acid [6,42]. On the contrary, the interference of saccharides is very significant in the bacterial biosensor: fructose 64%, glucose 63%, galactose 28%, and lactose 18% of the response to ascorbic acid [6].

It is interesting to compare various lactate cell-based biosensors from the point of view of their selectivity. The biosensor with the yeast *Hansenula anomala* responds to glucose and pyruvate, if oxygen uptake is measured [121,150]. If the electron transport mediator is used, the yeast biosensor is at first entirely specific. However, after a week-long operation, the interference of a great number of various compounds starts to rise, as seen in Table 6.3 [132]. The erythrocyte lactate biosensor responds not only to lactate, but also slightly to malate, and it has another disadvantage—a long response time [7]. The latter two biosensors use platinum anode as a transducer; for this reason, reducing substances from the sample can interfere with the measurement. Finally, the biosensor with the cells of *Escherichia coli* gains the selectivity to lactate only after a complicated combination of procedures—see Table 6.5 [99].

The selectivity of biosensors for urea determination is inconsistent as well. The hybrid biosensor with urease and nitrifying bacteria is entirely selective [15]; the tissue biosensor using urease activity in Jack bean may respond to some amino acids, but the measured signal is always less than 6% of that caused by urea [121]. The selectivity of urea microbe biosensors with *Proteus mirabilis* is the worst: if an ammonia electrode is used for detection, tryptophane and phenylalanine strongly interfere [91], while in the detection of carbon dioxide production, other than nitrogen-containing compounds – inositol and phenol – can also interfere [81]. With regard to the fact that interfering substances are not at all present in blood or only in concentrations incomparably less than that of urea, all of the cell-based biosensors described above can be used for urea determination in this biological fluid.

If we compare asparagine interference with glutamine determination, we find out that the biosensor with a slice of porcine kidney does not respond to asparagine at all [13], the microbial electrode with *Sarcina flava* responds to asparagine much less than to glutamine [13], and when we use the petal of a magnolia as a bioreceptor, both of these amino acids give the same signal [120]. It can be explained as follows: animal glutaminase (E.C. 3.5.1.2) is specific for glutamine deamination. On the contrary, the analogic enzyme known from bacterial systems and plant tissue catalyzes the hydrolysis of both glutamine and asparagine and thus can be better named glutamine-(asparagine-)ase, E.C. 3.5.1.38.

The results of interference studies in glucose cell-based biosensors are also very interesting. As seen from Table 6.7, only the biosensors with the cells of *Pseudomonas fluorescens* or human erythrocytes are genuine glucose biosensors, because interference of other sugars is negligible [9,48]. The biosensors with *Aspergillus niger* [152] or *Gluconobacter oxidans* [29] can be used if maltose is not present in analyzed samples. All other types of "glucose biosensors" also respond to other monosaccharides and some disaccharides. As most of them were prepared with cells that had been cultivated in a glucose-rich medium, it is presumable that their selectivity will gradually grow worse as they are used. It appears to be more convenient to use the term biosensors for estimating assimilable [125], or reducing sugars [75].

Mono- and polyphenoloxidases are widely distributed among different plant tissues and yeast species. Since each individual enzyme tends to catalyze the oxidation of one particular phenolic substrate more readily than others [3,19,104,131], the biosensors with different cells or tissues can serve for more or less selective determination of various phenolic compounds as it was mentioned in Section 5.1.4 and summarized in Table 5.2.

The comparison of other biosensor groups would be possible, for example, for the detection of pyruvate, oxalate, phenylalanine, tryptophane, ammonia, arginine, sucrose, methanol, or ethanol (see Table A.1). If more than one biosensor for the determination of the same substrate exists, the biosensor with the best selectivity is marked in that table.

TABLE 6.7. *Relative Response of Glucose Microbial Biosensors to Some Other Sugars; Response to Glucose of the Same Concentration Equals 100%.*

Microbial Cells	Measured Product	Relative Response (%)						Ref.
		Fructose	Galactose	Mannose	Sucrose	Maltose	Lactose	
Pseudomonas fluorescens	O_2	3.9	8.9	4.0	3.6	0	0	[48]
Aspergillus niger	O_2	0	0	0	0	20.0	0	[150]
Gluconobacter oxidans	H^+	0	9.0	0	0	20.0	0	[29]
Hansenula anomala	H^+	68.0	11.5	73.7	0	36.6	0	[101]
Bacillus subtilis	O_2	–	–	–	–	20.9	–	[50]
Saccharomyces cerevisiae	O_2, H^+	75	–	–	160	60	0	[49]
Brevibacterium lactofermentum	O_2	80	–	–	92	–	–	[125]
Streptococcus mutans	H^+	100	100	100	0	0	0	[20]
Bacteria from a dental plaque	H^+	100	0	100	0	0	0	[75]

6.16 CHOOSING A SUITABLE MODE OF THE MEASUREMENT

The biosensor response to the interfering substance can sometimes differ from its response to the substrate from a chronolgical point of view. It could be caused by different rates of the substrate and interferant diffusion through the membrane covering the cell layer or through the cell membrane itself. Another cause can be the unequal rates of metabolism for these two substances. If the difference between response times for the substrate and the interfering substance is great enough, it may be used for the selectivity enhancement of the biosensor.

Thus, the response of the amperometric biosensor with the cells of *Gluconobacter suboxidans* to ethanol is very quick, and the steady state is reached within 30 s. On the other hand, the response of the same biosensor to glucose appears slowly, and the steady-state current was attained only 15 min after adding glucose to the solution. The researchers explain this by a more deeply located glucose dehydrogenase in the cytoplasmatic membrane. If we register the current 30 s after the sample addition, ethanol is determined almost exclusively and glucose interference is negligible (Figure 6.6) [43].

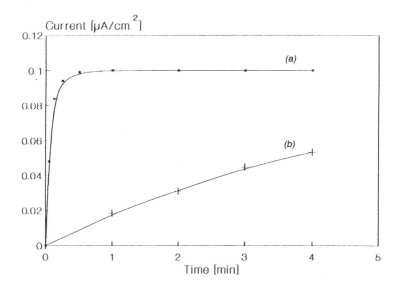

FIGURE 6.6. Current-time curves for the oxidation of ethanol (a) and glucose (b) at the electrode with *Gluconobacter suboxidans* (concentration of both substrates 0.1 mmol/l). (Adapted after Ikeda, T., K. Matsuyama, D. Kobayashi, and F. Matsuhita. 1992. *Biosci. Biotech. Biochem.*, 56(8):1359–1360. With permission.)

The principle of selectivity improvement of the biosensor with a rabbit muscle slice is similar. This biosensor is used for adenosine monophosphate (AMP) determination. Its response to this compound is three to five times quicker than to adenosine diphosphate (ADP). Equivalent potentials are measured only at an ADP/AMP concentration ratio of about fifty; therefore, a significant interference of ADP will occur only in the presence of ADP concentrations approaching the ADP/AMP ratio given above [107].

Glucose interferes with inorganic phosphate determination involving a hybrid electrode that contains a potato slice and glucose oxidase. Glucose is the product derived from the spliting of glucose-6-phosphate with acid phosphatase in potato and, at the same time, the substrate of the next enzyme – glucose oxidase. Glucose interference can be eliminated in two different ways. One possibility is to first add the analyzed material with phosphates and glucose (e.g., urine of diabetic patients), and only after the electrode signal has reached the steady state, then add the substrate – glucose-6-phosphate [114,115]. Other researchers have eliminated glucose interference by using glucose-6-phosphate concentrations ten times higher than the concentrations used by the authors cited above. This procedure seems to be more simple, but also more expensive [118].

Glucose or fructose also interferes with sucrose determination using invertase and *Zymomonas mobilis* cells in a hybrid biosensor – see Figure 6.2. Glucose-fructose oxidoreductase catalyzes conversion of equimolar amounts of glucose and fructose – the products of sucrose hydrolysis. This biosensor has a glass electrode as a transducer, which registers the fall in pH caused by produced gluconic acid. If glucose or fructose are present in the analyzed solution, the initial rate of response change is accelerated. On the other hand, it was found that the response value at a steady state is determined by the substrate of lower concentration and, therefore, by using the steady-state mode of measurement, interference of glucose or fructose is eliminated. However, if both of these sugars exist simultaneously in a sucrose sample, the interference is not avoided by this measurement mode; pretreatment of the sample with glucose removal is necessary in this case – see Section 6.6 [112].

As previously shown, reducing substances, primarily ascorbic and uric acids, interfere with all amperometric measurements that are based on the registration of the current arising during oxidation of the enzyme reaction product on the anode. Besides the possibilities that were discussed in Section 6.5, the following way to eliminate this interference is possible: to change the anode with the measurement on the cathode. If hydrogen peroxide production is examined in the glucose oxidase catalyzed reaction, ascorbic and uric acid interference is established. [113]. The same problem arises if another electron acceptor is used instead of oxygen [2]. But in another situation, if the same reaction is controlled as the oxygen concentration decreases, this interference type cannot be observed; the oxygen electrode is plugged in as the cathode, and in addition, it is covered with a membrane that is impermeable for ionized interfering substances [115,118].

Another possibility is to coimmobilize peroxidase with the system that uses glucose oxidase; hydrogen peroxide is reduced with potassium hexacyanoferrate(II), and the resulting hexacyanoferrate(III) is detected amperometrically on the cathode; neither ascorbic nor uric acid can interfere [152]

$$\text{Glucose} + O_2 \xrightarrow{\text{glucose oxidase}} \delta\text{-gluconolactone} + H_2O_2$$

$$H_2O_2 + 2\ Fe(CN)_6^{4-} + 2H^+ \xrightarrow{\text{peroxidase}} 2\ Fe(CN)_6^{3-} + 2H_2O$$

Dopamine and other catecholamines can be determined by a direct oxidation on the anode, but again, with a strong interference of ascorbic acid. If a tissue electrode with a banana pulp [18,19,154] or spinach leaf [131] is used, dopamine is oxidized in the cells to dopamine quinone. This enzyme reaction can be examined without ascorbic acid interference as oxygen consumption during dopamine oxidation, or amperometrically or voltammetrically as dopamine quinone reduction on a special electrode [18,19]. In the latter method, a slight interference of ascorbic acid could still be observed; this substance reduced dopamine quinone, and the biosensor response to domapine decreased by 10–20% [19].

6.17 USE OF A BLANK TEST

If the influence of interfering substances cannot be eliminated with any of the methods given so far, one more possibility exists: using a two-electrode system in which one of the electrodes represents a blank test. Its signal is then subtracted from the signal of the proper measuring electrode with active cells.

This method was used, for example, in the case of the lactate biosensor with the cells of *Hansenula anomala* immobilized in an acetylcellulose membrane on the surface of a platinum anode. The blank value is obtained from the electrode that was constructed in the same way as the active electrode, but with the cells treated with oxalate, which is known to be an irreversible inhibitor of yeast lactate dehydrogenase [46].

The biosensor for tryptophane determination uses a multi-step oxidative degradation of this amino acid in the cells of *Pseudomonas fluorescens*, immobilized on the surface of an oxygen electrode. Interfering substances can be divided into two groups:

(1) Intermediate substrates of multi-enzyme tryptophane oxidation, as L-kynurenine, anthranilic acid, or L-alanine
(2) Other amino acids, glucose, fructose, and uric acid

Synthesis induction of tryptophane-converting enzymes improves the biosensor selectivity only with respect to the substances of group (2). That is why it is necessary to subtract the signal that is produced with the electrode, which was prepared with the cells of the same microbial strain cultured in a tryptophane-free medium [96].

Lactobacillus fermenti cannot grow without thiamin; therefore, it was used for the estimation of this vitamin – see Section 6.2 [23]. If the yeast *Saccharomyces cerevisiae* is used for the same purpose, we must keep in mind that the cells of this yeast species can also grow without thiamin, although its addition to the culture medium will accelerate the cell growth considerably. The use of a blank is essential for this biosensor function. The yeast membrane is prepared with the cells immobilized in calcium alginate gel. The thiamin assay is a differential procedure that relies on the response of the yeast electrode before and after incubation in a thiamin-containing sample. The respiration intensity of the cell membrane during glucose assimilation is measured by an oxygen electrode [60].

Elimination of the interference of different pH values in urine samples in glycosuria determination, with the yeast biosensor containing the cells of *Hansenula anomala* in calcium alginate gel on the surface of a glass electrode, is also possible only with a blank electrode. This electrode is prepared in the same way as the measuring electrode except with the use of yeast cells, the glycolytic system of which was thermoinactivated. The fall in pH values, which is registered by the active electrode, must be corrected by the change of a signal, produced with a blank electrode [101].

The lactate biosensor based on lactate dehydrogenase activity of human erythrocytes uses hexacyanoferrate(III) and phenazine methosulfate as mediators of electron transport and amperometric detection of produced hexacyanoferrate(II) on the platinum anode (Figure 6.7). Since other reducing substances from biological material could also be oxidized on the anode, their interference was eliminated in the following way. The analyzed material was added to the working buffer with electron transfer mediators, but without coenzyme NAD^+. Within 2–3 min, the current reached the steady value proportional to the concentration of reducing substances in the sample. Only then, was coenzyme NAD^+ added, and the current increase

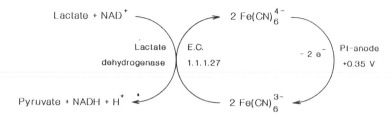

FIGURE 6.7. Principle of lactate determination with the erythrocyte-based biosensor.

that followed had already been caused by lactate oxidation. The influence of all reducing substances could be eliminated by this procedure; on the other hand, it was unable to eliminate interference of those compounds that are metabolized within the cells in a similar way as lactate, for example, malate [7].

Table 6.8 summarizes the ways to eliminate the interference of reducing substances during amperometric measurements on an anode, which were mentioned in this and some previous sections of this chapter.

6.18 ABSENCE OF INTERFERING SUBSTANCES IN THE ANALYZED SAMPLE

Although the cell-based biosensor is not quite selective, even when all the methods for its selectivity improvement have been employed, it can still sometimes be used in practice — for the analysis of those samples in which the interfering substance is absent. If we pass the analysis of monocomponental solutions, where all biosensors can be used — even those which are the least selective — the following examples illustrate the successful use of the less selective biosensors for the analysis of biological material.

The hybrid biosensor with the cells of *Escherichia coli* and glucose oxidase can be used for the determination of lactose concentration in milk products, since interfering glucose is absent in milk [116]. The biosensor for the determination of aspartame responds to glucose even three times higher than it does to aspartame. Nevertheless, it was successfully used for the determination of this artificial sweetener in drinks just because they do not contain glucose [147].

The biosensor with the yeast *Hansenula anomala* responds not only to glucose, but also to other sugars like mannose, fructose, maltose, and galactose. Regardless, it can be used for urine analysis in diabetic patients because the interfering sugars, with the exception of some heritable metabolic disorders that are very rare, cannot be found in urine [101]. Three of

TABLE 6.8. *Possible Ways of Elimination of Reducing Substances Interference during Amperometric Measurements on Anode.*

Way of Interference Elimination	References	Section Number
Reducing substance removal from the sample (oxidation with FeCl₃ in a solution or by hydrogen peroxide and peroxidase in a membrane)	[119] [139]	6.5
Hindrance of reducing substance diffusion to the anode		
Coimmobilization of ascorbate oxidase with the cells	[138]	6.5
Use of an acetylcellulose permselective membrane covering the transducer	[134,139]	
Use of a gas-permeable teflon membrane covering the transducer	[85]	
Subtraction of a blank value		
Use of the second electrode with inactivated cells	[46]	6.17
Successive addition of reagents to the active electrode with the cells	[7]	
Conversion of the measurement mode to reduction on cathode		
Measuring oxygen consumption instead of hydrogen peroxide production	[115,118]	6.16
Coimmobilization of peroxidase with hexacyanoferrate(II) addition to the sample	[152]	
Conversion of the substrate to a reducible substance in the cells	[18,19]	
High degree of enzyme synthesis induction in the cells (the signal produced by the substrate conversion is incomparably higher than that produced by the interferant)	[132]	6.8

the cell-based biosensors for urea determination are not wholly specific for this substrate – see Section 6.15. As in both serum and urine, the concentration of potentially interfering substances is incomparably lower than the concentration of urea, these biosensors can be used for the measurement of urea concentration in biological fluids, with the exception of the cases with elevated glucose concentration, when the biosensor with the cells of *Proteus mirabilis* and a carbon dioxide electrode as a transducer is not convenient [84].

Also, both biosensors using a cucumber or yellow squash slice are useable in practice. It is important to mention that the biosensor for ascorbic acid analysis responds with 80% intensity to isoascorbic acid as well, but this compound is not present in juices and drinks [6,42]. Pyruvate would interfere in glutamate determination (it gives 15.6% of the biosensor response to glutamate), but it is also not common in the analyzed material (i.e., in fermentation broths) [31].

In phosphate determination with the hybrid biosensor using a potato slice and glucose oxidase, fluorides, molybdates, and nitrates interfere; they also inhibit acid phosphatase in this plant tissue. These anions cannot interfere in urine in significant concentrations [114,115].

The biosensor for methanol determination with unidentified bacteria responds to ethanol with the same intensity [52]. The microbial biosensor with the cells of *Trichosporon brassicae* is not very selective for acetic acid – a decrease in oxygen concentration can also be caused by the metabolization of ethanol, propionic acid, or butyric acid [53]. In spite of these observations, both biosensors were successfully used for the determination of methanol and acetic acid in the fermentation broths in such processes where interfering substances are not produced.

The biosensor with the cell of *Thiobacillus ferrooxidans* on the surface of an oxygen electrode can be used for iron determination in mine effluents and acidic extracts of sulfidic minerals containing a number of metals along with iron; the presence of potentially interfering cations, such as U^{4+}, Cu^+, and Sn^{2+} in real solutions, is unlikely [102].

6.19 UNSELECTIVITY IS INTENDED

Up to this point, we have discussed the possibilities of how to improve insufficient biosensor selectivity with the aim of obtaining a biosensor that would respond exclusively, or at any rate, largely to one substance. On the contrary, we can meet the requirement for the biosensor to respond to the greatest number of metabolites possible.

Among these biosensors, the largest group is represented by the biosensors used for estimating BOD in waste waters. The biosensors of this type use bacterial or yeast cells of defined strains, in mixtures isolated from activated sludges, or from soil. These microbes are cultivated in rich nutritious media so that the cells can metabolize the greatest possible number of various substrates. A Clark oxygen electrode is the most common transducer; the decrease in oxygen partial pressure in the nearest environs of the cells is proportional to the degree of organic water pollution. The solution with equal concentrations of glucose and glutamic acid is usually used as a standard [56–59]. Table 6.9 shows the example of the BOD biosensor with the cells of *Trichosporon cutaneum* compared with the classical five-day method of BOD estimation. The biosensor unselectivity can be seen from the table.

Some respiratory biosensors are another example where the selectivity is not necessary. The principle of their function was described in Section 2.3.2. The unselectivity of this system is manifested not only during microbe cultivation in a rich medium, but also with respect to the determined substance. This is to say that the biosensor is sensitive to the whole group of compounds that inhibit the growths and, thus, the respiration of microbial cells. The same biosensor could be used for the estimation of (1) various aminoglycosidic antibiotics [62,63], (2) other biosensors for the detection of polyene antimycotic drugs [64,65], (3) various tetracyclines [24],

TABLE 6.9. Relative Response of the Yeast Biosensor with Trichosporon cutaneum *to Organic Compounds and Its Comparison with the Five-Day Method of BOD Determination; Response to Glucose Equals 100%.*

	Biosensor Response (%)	Five-Day Method of BOD Determination (%)
Ethanol	403	197
Acetic acid	246	248
Glucose	100	100
Lactic acid	100	74
Glutamate	97	96
Fructose	75	67
Glycerol	71	62
Glycine	63	74
Sucrose	50	51
Histidine	49	57
Citric acid	24	38
Soluble starch	10	7
Lactose	8	9

Adapted after Hikuma, M., H. Suzuki, T. Yasuda, I. Karube, and S. Suzuki. 1979. *Europ. J. Appl. Microbiol. Biotenchnol.*, 8:289–297. With permission.

or (4) mutagens [66]. The respiratory biosensor with human fibroblasts or mouse leukemia cells was used for the screening of antitumor drugs [10]. Because it is known which drug from the whole group the patient uses and, thus, which compound should be determined in biological material, the unselectivity is not disadvantageous; on the contrary, it enables the use of one cell type for the analysis of a number of drugs or compounds with similar action. This is usually impossible with most immunochemical methods where the antibody selectivity is greater; those methods can be used for the detection of a lower number of compounds with a similar chemical structure.

CHAPTER 7

Practical Use of Cell-Based Biosensors

The practical use of cell-based biosensors is limited, for the most part, by three conditions. The first is to reach a sufficient selectivity for a given analytical purpose. The possibilities of selectivity improvement and the evaluation of these methods was discussed in the previous chapter. The other two conditions are the reasonably short response time and the long-term stability of the biosensor. While stability of most cell-based biosensors is long enough, the response time is sometimes so long that the biosensor could not be used for measurements in a greater series.

Although almost all researchers showed the possibility of practical use of their biosensor, only several of them really verified this possibility and compared the use of the biosensor with other analytical methods. This situation is summarized in the following sections.

7.1 USE IN CLINICAL CHEMISTRY

Many cell-based biosensors were successfully used for measurements of various substrates in blood, blood serum, urine, or cerebrospinal fluid of patients.

Thus, for example, the results obtained by the lactate cell-based biosensor with the yeast *Hansenula anomala*, were favourably comparable with routine spectrophotometric UV-test (correlation coefficient $r = 0.976$, Figure 7.1) and the results obtained with the enzyme electrode containing an isolated yeast lactate dehydrogenase ($r = 0.990$); blood plasma and whole blood were used as a biological material. A 2–3 min response time, a good reproducibility expressed as a variation coefficient in a series within 2.31 and 3.72%, and a sufficient long-term stability are the properties supporting

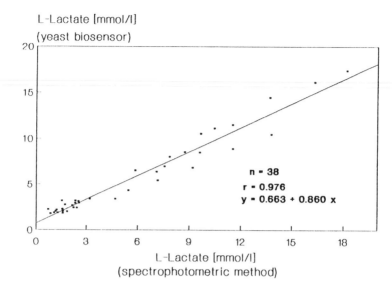

FIGURE 7.1. Comparison of a yeast lactate biosensor with *Hansenula anomala* and a spectrophotometric UV-test for lactate; blood plasma samples were used for measurements. (Reprinted from Racek, J. and J. Musil. 1987. *Clin. Chim. Acta*, 162(2):129–139. With permission of Elsevier Science Publishers BV.)

the use of this biosensor in practice [45,46]. The lactate biosensor with human erythrocytes also gave results practically identical to the UV-test ($r = 0.995$) if lactate concentration in whole blood was measured; its practical use is, however, limited by a slow response [7].

All cell-based biosensors for urea determination were also used in laboratory practice: the biosensor with the cells of *Proteus mirabilis* and the detection of carbon dioxide for urine and whole blood analysis [83], with the same cells except ammonia detection for urine analysis [93], the biosensor based on immobilized Jack bean tissue and a conductivity detection for serum analysis [25], and the hybrid biosensor with urease and nitrifying bacteria was tested for the measurement of urea concentration in urine samples [15]. In all of these cases a good correlation with the spectrophotometric method was found with correlation coefficients within the range of 0.970–0.987.

The cell biosensor with *Nocardia erythropolis* was tested in measuring cholesterol in sera diluted ten times. With a glucose concentration within the physiological range, no interfering compounds were found, and the reproducibility of 2–7% was sufficient [78]. Blood serum was also used for measuring lysozyme concentration with the biosensor based on the cells of

Micrococcus lysodeicticus loaded with trimethylphenylammonium ion [71], or for glutamine quantification with the cells of *Sarcina flava* on the surface of an ammonia electrode [88]. Glutamine in cerebrospinal fluid was estimated with the tissue biosensor using a porcine kidney slice as a receptor [106]. The hybrid biosensor of a reactor type with the cell suspension of *Leuconostoc mesenteroides* and the lactate enzyme electrode was used for phenylalanine determination in twenty human blood sera samples; the results were compared with phenylalanine determination that was performed on an automatic amino acid analyzer having a correlation coefficient of 0.91 [21].

Oxalates in urine samples were determined with the biosensor using an acetone-treated banana skin with a relative error of 2.5% [119]. The hybrid biosensor with a potato slice and glucose oxidase was used for inorganic phosphate determination in urine, serum, and pharmaceutical products; it was found to have a very good reproducibility (variation coefficient within the range of 0.9–6.6%) and results comparable with the photometric method [114,115,118].

The respiration biosensor with the cells of *Escherichia coli* and a carbon dioxide electrode as a transducer was used for measuring gentamicine and other aminoglycosides in the sera of patients. The results were available within 2 hr in comparison with an 18–20-hr period necessary for the conventional tests [63].

Finally, both cell-based biosensor types for hydrogen peroxide determination were used in a final phase of heterogenous immunoassay; peroxidase activity was estimated on the basis of its competition for hydrogen peroxide with catalase in a slice of bovine liver tissue [155], or in human erythrocytes [156], on the surface of an oxygen electrode. The results were comparable with those obtained with a classical photometric detection of peroxidase activity, but the length of time necessary for the electrochemical method can be counted as a disadvantage.

7.2 USE IN FOOD ANALYSIS

In theory, cell-based biosensors could be used in analyzing the food composition of proteins, saccharides, amino acids, vitamins, or the compounds that are artificially added to food such as artificial sweeteners, preserving agents, etc. Nevertheless, in practice only several cell-based biosensors were used for this purpose.

The useability of the tissue biosensor with a yellow squash slice for ascorbic acid determination in fruit juices was verified on the basis of comparing the results with polarographic analysis [42]. The excellent selectivity of the hybrid electrode composed from coimmobilized invertase and *Zymomonas mobilis* cells, using a glass electrode as a transducer, was used in an analysis of drinks sweetened with sucrose [112]. Lactose in milk products was determined with another hybrid biosensor, this time with the cells of *Escherichia coli* and glucose oxidase; this application utilizes the fact that glucose, otherwise a strongly interfering substance, is absent in these products [116]. Similarly, sucrose in various drinks was determined with a hybrid biosensor using *Saccharomyces cerevisiae* and glucose oxidase; the results were compared with the results obtained by a three-enzyme electrode [141].

Short-chain fatty acids in milk were detected with a microbial electrode based on the cells of *Arthrobacter nicotiana* fitted on the surface of an oxygen electrode by means of a dialysis membrane. This method was found to have a very good correspondence with gas chromatography [129].

7.3 USE IN CONTROL OF FERMENTATION PROCESSES

The possibility of using the cell-based biosensors in this field is great. Since the cells used as a receptor often respond to more compounds, it is necessary to improve the biosensor selectivity or to use it only in those cases when we are sure that interfering substances cannot be produced [51]. At other times, the unselectivity is useful, for example, if we want to examine the content of assimilable sugars in fermentation broth regardless of what their relative amounts are. Thus, the assimilable sugars – glucose, fructose, and mannose – in fermentation broth were measured with the biosensor using the cells of *Brevibacterium lactofermentum* [125].

The biosensor based on the transformation of formic acid in the cells of *Clostridium butyricum* with amperometric detection of produced gaseous hydrogen was used for the determination of this organic acid in fermentation broth. The results were compared with those that were obtained by gas chromatography. Their correspondence was expressed by the correlation coefficient of 0.98 [136]. The biosensor based on the cells of *Trichosporon brassicae* on the surface of an oxygen electrode was successfully used for the determination of acetic acid in the fermentation broth of glutamic acid [52,53]. Ethanol concentration during production of beer, wine, or vinegar was examined by the same biosensor covered with a gas-permeable membrane. The biosensor was used for 2100 assays without losing its sensitivity. The results were again comparable to gas chromatography with a correlation coefficient of 0.98 [51,52].

7.4 USE IN ENVIRONMENTAL CONTROL

Practical applications of cell-based biosensors in this field are connected with the control of waste water pollution, expecially with organic substances. The method for the determination of biological oxygen demand as a criterion for organic water pollution in its classical form lasts five days; the use of biosensors reduced this time to several hours with the same results. The respiratory electrode with *Trichosporon cutaneum* was used for BOD estimation in untreated waste waters from a fermentation factory. Comparison of the results with the classical five-day method gave a correlation coefficient of 0.95. Table 6.8 compares the biosensor response to various organic compounds with the five-day method; in most cases, a good correspondence was found [54,100]. A good correlation in similar comparisons was described by other researchers who used the biosensor with bacteria from soil [26], thermophilic bacteria from hot springs [53], or bacteria from activated sludges [58] for the examination of waste waters. Better results were found in the case of pollution with low molecular compounds; on the other hand, the examination of water polluted with organic macromolecules or large organic particles gave lower results if the biosensor was used [57]. This is explained by an inaccessibility of these particles for the cells since the cells were immobilized within a membrane and were often covered with a dialysis membrane as well [54,57,58].

Individual compounds in waste waters were also examined. The biosensor with nitrifying bacteria was used for ammonia determination in waste water from a fermentation factory. A good correspondence with a conventional method was given by a correlation coefficient of 0.90 [11,88,100]. Phenol was estimated with a sufficient selectivity in waste water samples with the biosensor containing the cells of *Trichosporon cutaneum* [41]. The selectivity for phenol was achieved in this yeast strain during cultivation of the yeast cells in a phenol-rich medium. In another case, the same yeast species was used for the BOD biosensor construction, only after cultivation in a medium of complex composition with many different nutrients [51,98].

Inorganic compounds can also be estimated by cell-based biosensors. A hybrid biosensor was used for inorganic phosphate determination in water. The biosensor responded not only to phosphates, but also to polyphosphates that could be found in waste waters as well. Nitrates interfered with this estimation [114,115].

Heavy metals in the environment could be estimated with a biosensor, based on their uptake by lichen thalli followed by voltammetric detection [4].

Gaseous compounds in the atmosphere can also be registered with a sufficient sensitivity and excellent selectivity by microbial biosensors. The biosensor for methane determination uses microbial cells of *Methylomonas flagellata*; the results were compared with the measurement of methane concentration by gas chromatography with a correlation coefficient of 0.97 [22,92]. Nitrifying bacteria were used for the selective detection of nitrogen dioxide; the results obtained with the biosensor were practically identical to those where a conventional method was used [93].

CHAPTER 8

Conclusions and Future Prospects

Enzyme electrodes were the first biosensors constructed. Only later on were other biosensing receptors used (whole cells, along with recently recognized various immunomolecules or isolated cell receptors), making it possible to detect new types of compounds. Transducers used in biosensor construction developed from classical amperometric or potentiometric electrodes to ion-sensitive field-effect transistors, optical transducers, and others.

The accessibility of biosensors is given primarily by their serial production. Many biosensors form the basis of commercially available analyzers that can be used in medicine, the food industry, or biotechnology. More than half of these analyzers are intended for glucose analysis, but analyzers for the determination of lactate, uric acid, ethanol, and several other compounds also exist [161]. All of these commercially available biosensors are based on enzyme electrodes with an isolated enzyme that is immobilized in a membrane on the transducer surface.

Although the possibility of using whole cells as a bioreceptor has been known for about fifteen years and dozens of various cell-based biosensors have been constructed, they are—with few exceptions—prepared only in laboratories, and their routine use, facilitated by possible serial production, remains only a wish. There are several reasons for this. Advantages of cell-based biosensors such as their easy construction without previous enzyme isolation, purification, and immobilization (which keeps the cost down) is lost due to the serial production and commercial availability of many enzyme biosensors, which is also cost effective. On the other hand, the main problem remains—it is, in many cases, insufficient selectivity of cell-based biosensors in comparison with analogical enzyme electrodes. It is necessary to take into account their use in analysis of biological fluids, the composition of which is complex; the presence of a great number of potentially interfering substances in those samples can be expected. In addition, the response of cell-based biosensors is sometimes slower and fluctuates from day to day, depending on the status or growth of the cells on the transducer surface. The ultimate purpose of this book is to show the complexity of problems linked with cell-based biosensors, especially with their selectivity, and to solve the problems that hinder these biosensors in routine practice. A broad interdisciplinary cooperation and collaboration of biochemists, organic chemists, physical chemists, biologists, and microbiologists is necessary for new biosensor development, among which cell-based biosensors can play an important role. Their collaboration is also a precondition for preparing standard cell suspensions that would be stable for a long time and, above all, commercially available so that the sensing part of the cell-based biosensor could be renewed whenever necessary, keeping all of the important biosensor properties unchanged.

It can be assumed that in the near future, thanks to the cooperation of scientists working in various fields of chemistry and biology, new cell types will be applied for biosensor construction, thus enabling them to be used for the analysis of new varieties of biomolecules. These less common cell types could include erythrocytes, leucocytes, and the cells isolated from tissues, lichens or various mushrooms as mentioned in previous chapters. Also, other tissue classes — those from insects or aquatic plants — have been investigated.

The only kind of cell-based biosensors that scored a greater use in practice are respiratory electrodes. It may be easily explained: in this biosensor type no analogy with enzyme electrodes exists; they cannot be replaced with any type of enzyme electrodes because it is necessary to use living cells for their function. The function of respiratory electrodes is inseparably linked to vital functions such as respiration or keeping the cell integrity. Great progress of cell-based biosensors can be expected in this field alone. Respiration electrodes with sensitive cells can be used in the detection and the quantification of antibiotics, antitumor drugs, mutagens, and other harmful substances. The effect of these compounds on the cells is usually irreversible, and that is why in most of these biosensors, the cell-based receptor must be renewed after each measurement, which makes their use in continuous monitoring of harmful substances in waste waters or in the atmosphere impossible. Nevertheless, the use of cell-based biosensors for this purpose represents a great contribution in comparison with time-consuming classical methods. The other possibility is the use of respiratory electrodes for continuous monitoring of water pollution with organic compounds (as BOD), which has already been used not only in experiments, but also in routine practice. Some other biosensors based on immobilized microbes on the surface of an oxygen electrode are reuseable, although they are not genuine respiratory electrodes; they can be applied to the detection of individual organic compounds [41,163].

In conclusion, it may be said that cell-based biosensors have their place among other biosensor types. Although they cannot replace enzyme electrodes, they can complement their analytical use in special indications due to different properties. Serial production and commercial availability of cell-based biosensors would certainly promote their practical use.

In conclusion, a tabular survey of cell-based biosensors is given with special respect to their selectivity (Table A.1). The biosensors are arranged in alphabetical order according to the substrates for the determination of which they were proposed.

The interference type is specified by the numbers that correspond to the itemization in Chapter 5 into its sections. Similarly, the way of selectivity improvement – if it is mentioned by the researchers – is specified by the number corresponding with the itemization in Chapter 6.

The selectivity degree (after all methods of selectivity improvement were applied) is classified according to the following criteria:

(1) The biosensor is entirely selective
(2) Selectivity-sufficient
(3) Selectivity-sufficient only in definite cases
(4) Selectivity-poor
(5) Selectivity-inconvenient
(6) The biosensor unselectivity intended

TABLE A.1. Various Cell-Based Biosensors with Respect to Their Selectivity; Abbreviations Used:
DCPIP—2,6-Dichlorphenolindophenol, TMPA⁺—Trimethylphenylammonium Ion, X²⁺—Divalent Cation of Heavy Metal.

Substrate	Cell Type	Detected Substance	Interference Type	Method of Selectivity Improvement	Selectivity Degree	References
Acetic acid	Trichosporon brassicae	O_2	1.4,2.2	18	3	[52,53]
Adenosine	Mouse small intestine mucosal cells	NH_3	2.1,2.2	9,10	1	[32]
Adenosine 5'-phosphate	Rabbit muscle	NH_3	2.1, 2.2	10,16	2	[107]
Adiuretine	Toad bladder	Na^+	1.4	–	3	[72]
Aminoglycosides	Escherichia coli	CO_2	1.4	18	2	[63]
	Escherichia coli	O_2	1.4	18	2	[62]
α-Amylase	Bacillus subtilis	O_2	–	8	1	[39]
	Bacillus subtilis + glucoamylase	O_2	–	8,15	1	[39]
Ammonia	Nitrosomonas europaea or nitrifying bacteria	O_2	2.2, 2.3	8,13	2	[89]
	Nitrifying bacteria	O_2	–	–	–	[52]
	Nitrosomonas sp. + Nitrobacter sp.	O_2	2.3	6,13,15	1	[11,98]
Antitumor drugs	Mouse leukemia cells	O_2	–	–	2	[10]
	Human foreskin fibroblasts	O_2	–	–	2	[10
Arginine	Streptococcus lactis	NH_3	2.2	–	2	[120]
	Streptococcus faecium	NH_3	2.2, 2.3	13	2	[74,77]
	Bovine liver + urease	NH_3	–	13	–	[156]

TABLE A.1. *(continued)*.

Substrate	Cell Type	Detected Substance	Interference Type	Method of Selectivity Improvement	Selectivity Degree	References
Ascorbic acid	*Enterobacter agglomerans*	O_2	1.4, 2.2	8	5	[6]
	Yellow squash or cucumber fruit	O_2	1.4, 2.2	15, 18	2	[6,42]
Assimilable sugars	*Brevibacterium lactofermentum*	O_2	2.2	19	5	[125]
Asparagine	*Serratia marcescens*	NH_3	–	8	2	[95]
	Petal of magnolia	NH_3	1.4	–	2	[123]
Aspartame	*Bacillus subtilis*	O_2	1.5, 2.2	8, 18	2	[147]
Aspartate	*Bacterium cadaveris*	NH_3	2.1, 2.2	12	5	[87]
	Bacillus subtilis	O_2	2.2	8	4	[50]
Biological oxygen demand (BOD)	*Bacillus subtilis*	O_2	2.2	19	6	[57]
	Clostridium butyricum	H_2	2.2	19	6	[55]
	Hansenula anomala	O_2	2.2	8	5	[151]
	Trichosporon cutaneum	O_2	2.2	19	6	[54,55,98]
	Bacteria from soil	O_2	2.2, 2.3	19	6	[26,55]
	Bacteria from active sludges	O_2	2.2, 2.3	19	6	[58]
	Thermophilic bacteria	O_2	2.2	19	6	[56]
	Pseudomonas sp.	O_2	2.2	19	6	[59]

(continued)

TABLE A.1. (continued).

Substrate	Cell Type	Detected Substance	Interference Type	Method of Selectivity Improvement	Selectivity Degree	References
Carbon dioxide	Pseudomonas sp.	O_2	2.2	6, 8	2	[143]
	Chemoautotrophic thermophilic bacteria	O_2	2.2	8	2	[158]
Catechol	Eggplant fruit	o-quinone	1.4	16	2	[131]
Catecholamines	Spinach leaf	O_2	1.4, 2.2	–	3	[130]
Cephalosporines	Citrobacter freundii	H^+	0	–	1	[35]
Cholesterol	Nocardia erythropolis	O_2	2.2	7, 8	2	[78]
Creatinine	Creatininase + Nitrosomonas sp. + Nitrobacter sp.	O_2	0	1	1	[14]
Cysteine	Proteus morganii	H_2S	1.3, 1.4	9	5	[85]
	Cucumber leaf	NH_3	–	–	–	[105]
Dopamine	Banana pulp	dopamine quinone	1.2, 1.4	16	4	[18,19]
	Banana pulp	O_2	–	–	–	[154]
	Spinach leaf	dopamine quinone	1.4	15, 16	2	[16]
Ethanol	Acetobacter aceti	H^+	1.4	6, 9	2	[28]
	Acetobacter xylinum	O_2	1.5, 2.2	–	2	[1]
	Gluconobacter suboxidans	$Fe(CN)_6^{4-}$	2.2	16	–	[43]
	Pichia pinus 2468	H^+	1.5	3	2	[30]
	Saccharomyces cerevisiae	$Fe(CN)_6^{4-}$	–	–	–	[44]
	Trichosporon brassicae	O_2	0	6, 9, 15	1	[51,52]

TABLE A.1. (continued).

Substrate	Cell Type	Detected Substance	Interference Type	Method of Selectivity Improvement	Selectivity Degree	References
Fatty acids	Arthrobacter nicotiana	O_2	1.4	8	2	[129]
Formaldehyde	Hansenula polymorpha A3-11	H^+	0	3	1	[31]
Formic acid	Clostridium butyricum	H_2	0	4, 5, 6, 15	1	[135]
	Pseudomonas oxalaticus	CO_2	2.2	7, 8, 12	3	[73]
Fructose	Zymomonas mobilis	H^+	1.4	7, 8	2	[100]
Glucosamine-6-phosphate	Porcine kidney	NH_3	2.2	9	2	[110]
Glucose	Aspergillus niger	$Fe(CN)_6^{4-}$	—	7, 8	—	[2]
	Aspergillus niger	O_2	2.2	15, 18	2	[152]
	Bacillus subtilis	O_2	2.2	8	4	[50]
	Gluconobacter oxidans	H^+	2.2	15, 18	2	[29]
	Hansenula anomala	H^+	2.2	8	3	[101]
	Human erythrocytes	H^+	0	4, 15	1	[9]
	Pseudomonas fluorescens	O_2	2.2	8, 15	2	[48,159]
	Saccharomyces cerevisiae	O_2	2.2	8	5	[49]
	Saccharomyces cerevisiae	CO_2	2.2	8	5	[49]
Glutamate	Bacillus subtilis	O_2	2.2	8, 10	2	[144]
	Escherichia coli	CO_2	2.2	4, 7, 8, 11	2	[33]
	Yellow squash fruit	CO_2	2.2	18	2	[34]

(continued)

TABLE A.1. (continued).

Substrate	Cell Type	Detected Substance	Interference Type	Method of Selectivity Improvement	Selectivity Degree	References
Glutamine	Sarcina flava	NH_3	1.4, 2.2	12	2	[13,88,109]
		NH_3	2.2	10, 15	1	[109,133,157]
	Porcine kidney					[5,13,106]
	Petal of magnolia	NH_3	1.4	–	2	[123]
Glycerol-3-phosphate	Escherichia coli	O_2	2.2	8, 10	1	[99]
Guanine	Rabbit liver	NH_3	2.1, 2.2	10	1	[103]
Heavy metal ions	Various lichens	X^{2+}	–	–	2	[2]
Histidine	Pseudomonas sp.	NH_3	1.5, 2.2	8	4	[37]
Hydrogen peroxide	Bovine liver	O_2	1.2	7	2	[111,155]
	Human erythrocytes	O_2	1.2	–	2	[8,156]
	Tobacco callus	ferricinium	–	–	–	[162]
Iron (Fe^{2+})	Thiobacillus ferrooxidans	O_2	1.4	8, 18	1	[102]
D-Lactate	Escherichia coli	O_2	2.2	10	1	[99]
L-Lactate	Hansenula anomala	$Fe(CN)_6^{4-}$	2.2	8, 10	2	[45,132]
	Hansenula anomala	$Fe(CN)_6^{4-}$	1.3, 2.2	7, 8, 17	1	[46,47,76]
	Hansenula anomala	O_2	2.2	8	4	[121,151]
	Escherichia coli	O_2	2.2	8, 10	1	[99]
	Human erythrocytes	$Fe(CN)_6^{4-}$	1.3, 2.1	17	1	[7]

Substrate	Cell Type	Detected Substance	Interference Type	Method of Selectivity Improvement	Selectivity Degree	References
Lactose	Escherichia coli + glucose oxidase	O_2	1.5	8, 12, 18	3	[116]
Lysozyme	Micrococcus lysodeicticus	TMPA⁺	0	–	1	[71]
Malate	Escherichia coli	O_2	2.2	8, 10	1	[99]
Methane	Methylomonas flagellata	O_2	0	1	1	[22, 92]
Methanol	Hansenula polymorpha 34-19	H⁺	1.5	3	2	[30]
	Unidentified bacteria	O_2	1.4	6, 9, 18	3	[51,52]
Methylsulfate	Hyphomicrobium sp.	H⁺	2.2	8	3	[79]
Mutagens	Bacillus subtilis M45 (Rec −)	O_2	0	3	2	[66]
	Salmonella typhimurium TA100	O_2	0	2, 3	2	[135]
NAD⁺	NAD⁺ – nucleotidase + Escherichia coli	NH_3	2.2	10	2	[113]
NAD(P)H	Escherichia coli	O_2	2.2	7, 10	2	[99]
Nicotinic acid	Lactobacillus arabinosus	H⁺	0	2	1	[97]
Nitrate	Azotobacter vinelandii	NH_3	1.5, 2.2	8	5	[36]

(continued)

91

TABLE A.1. (continued).

Substrate	Cell Type	Detected Substance	Interference Type	Method of Selectivity Improvement	Selectivity Degree	References
Nitrilotriacetic acid	Pseudomonas sp.	NH_3	1.5, 2.2	8, 10	5	[86]
	Pseudomonas sp.	CO_2	1.5, 2.2	8, 10	5	[86]
Nitrogen dioxide	Nitrifying bacteria	O_2	—	1	1	[93]
Nystatine	Saccharomyces cerevisiae	O_2	—	—	2	[64,65]
	Saccharomyces cerevisiae	CO_2	—	—	2	[65]
	Saccharomyces cerevisiae	Rb^+	—	—	2	[70]
Oxalate	Ground beet stem	H_2O_2	1.3, 2.2	5	2	[17]
	Banana skin	H_2O_2	1.3	5, 15	1	[119]
	Banana skin	CO_2	—	—	1	[119]
Peptides	Bacillus subtilis	O_2	2.2	8	4	[40]
Phenol	Trichosporon cutaneum	O_2	1.4, 2.2	8	3	[41]
	Fruit-body of Agaricus bisporus	O_2	1.4, 2.2	10, 15	3	[3]
Phenylalanine	Proteus vulgaris	NH_3	2.2	—	5	[83]
	Proteus mirabilis	NH_3	2.2	—	5	[83]
	Leuconostoc mesenteroides + lactate oxidase	O_2	0	15	1	[21]

TABLE A.1. (continued).

Substrate	Cell Type	Detected Substance	Interference Type	Method of Selectivity Improvement	Selectivity Degree	References
Phosphate	Potato tuber + glucose oxidase	O_2	1.4, 1.5	16, 18	2	[115,118]
	Potato tuber + glucose oxidase	H_2O_2	1.4, 1.5	18	2	[114]
Proteases	Bacillus subtilis	O_2	–	8	1	[40]
Proline	Pseudomonas sp.	O_2	2.2	8	2	[145]
Pyruvate	Streptococcus faecium	CO_2	2.2	10	3	[82]
	Escherichia coli	O_2	2.2	7, 10	–	[99]
	Corn kernel	CO_2	–	–	–	[108]
Reducing sugars	Bacteria from dental plaque	H^+	2.2	7, 19	3	[75]
	Streptococcus mutans	H^+	2.2	8	3	[20]
Serine	Clostridium acidiurici	NH_3	2.2	12	3	[80]
Steroid hormones	Nocardia opaca	DCPIP	1.4	8	4	[128]
Sucrose	Invertase + Zymomonas mobilis	H^+	1.5	6, 7, 8, 16	2	[112]
	Saccharomyces cerevisiae + glucose oxidase	O_2	1.5	7	2	[142]
Succinate	Escherichia coli	O_2	2.2	8, 10	2	[99]

(continued)

93

TABLE A.1. (continued.)

Substrate	Cell Type	Detected Substance	Interference Type	Method of Selectivity Improvement	Selectivity Degree	References
Sulfite	Thiobacillus thioparus	O_2	2.2	8	2	[122]
Tetracyclines	Escherichia coli	CO_2	1.5	18	2	[24]
Thiamin	Lactobacillus fermenti	Reductive substances	0	2, 15	1	[23]
	Saccharomyces cerevisiae	O_2	2.2	17	2	[60]
Tryptophane	Escherichia coli	NH_3	1.4, 2.2	8	5	[91]
	Pseudomonas fluorescens	O_2	1.4, 1.5, 2.2	8, 15, 17	3	[96]
Tyrosine	Aeromonas phenologenes	NH_3	2.2	8, 10	5	[81]
	Sugar beet root	O_2	1.4	–	3	[104]
Urea	Proteus mirabilis	NH_3	2.2	18	2	[94]
	Proteus mirabilis	CO_2	2.2	18	2	[84]
	Jack bean meal	NH_3	2.2	18	2	[124]
	Jack bean meal	NH_4^+	–	–	–	[25]
	Urease + Nitrosomonas sp. + Nitrobacter sp.	O_2	0	1, 15	1	[15]
Uric acid	Pichia membranaefaciens	CO_2	2.2	8	3	[133]

REFERENCES

1. Diviès, C. 1975. "Remarques sur l'oxydation de l'éthanol par une électrode micro-bienne' d'*Acetobacter xylinum*," *Ann. Microbiol, (Inst. Pasteur),* 126A:175–186.

2. Vincké, B. J., J. M. Kaufmann, M. J. Devleeschouwer, and G. J. Patriarche. 1984. "Nouveau modèle d'électrode enzymatique pour la détermination du glucose. Applications aux milieux biologiques," *Analusis,* 12(3):141–147.

3. Macholán, L. and L. Schánĕl. 1984. "Mushroom Tissue-Based Biocatalytic Electrode for Determination of Phenols," *Biologia (Bratislava),* 39(12):1191–1197.

4. Dempsey, E., M. R. Smyth, and D. H. S. Richardson. 1992. "Application of Lichen-Modified Carbon Paste Electrodes to the Voltammetric Determination of Metal Ions in Multi-Element and Speciation Studies," *Analyst,* 117(9):1467–1470.

5. Rechnitz, G. A., M. A. Arnold, and M. E. Meyerhoff. 1979. "Bio-Selective Mem-brane Electrode Using Tissue Slices," *Nature,* 278:466–467.

6. Vincké, B. J., M. J. Devleeschouwer, and G. J. Patriarche. 1985. "Determination de l'acide L-ascorbique a l'aide d'electrodes bacteriennes, tissulaires et enzymatiques," *Anal. Lett.,* 18(B 13):1593–1606.

7. Racek, J. 1987. "Lactate Biosensor Using Human Erythrocytes," *Anal. Chim. Acta,* 197:187–194.

8. Racek, J. and R. Petr. 1990. "Biosensor for Determination of Hydrogen Peroxide Based on Catalase Activity of Human Erythrocytes," *Anal. Chim. Acta,* 239:19–22.

9. Racek, J. 1993. "The Selectivity of Cell-Based Biosensors and Its Improvement," *Proceedings of the Symposium "Biosensorics in Central and Eastern Europe,"* March 22 and 23, 1993, Bochum, Federal Republic of Germany.

10. Li, X.-M., B. S. Liand, and H. Y. Wang. 1988. "Computer Aided Analysis for Bio-sensing and Screening," *Biotechnol. Bioeng.,* 31(2):250–256.

11. Karube, I., T. Okada, and S. Suzuki. 1981. "Amperometric Determination of Am-monia Gas with Immobilized Nitrifying Bacteria," *Anal. Chem.,* 53(12):1852–1854.

12. Racek, J. and J. Musil. 1990. "Possibilities of Lactate Determination by Cell Biosen-sors," *Proceedings of the Symposium on Bioanalytical Methods,* September 4–7, 1990, Prague, Czechoslovakia, pp. 36–38.

13. Arnold, M. A. and G. A. Rechnitz. 1980. "Comparison of Bacterial, Mitochondrial, Tissue and Enzyme Biocatalysts for Glutamine Selective Membrane Electrodes," *Anal. Chem.*, 52(8):1170–1174.

14. Kubo, I., I. Karube, and S. Suzuki. 1983. "Amperometric Determination of Creatinine with a Biosensor Based on Immobilized Creatininase and Nitrifying Bacteria," *Anal. Chim. Acta*, 151(1):371–376.

15. Okada, T., I. Karube, and S. Suzuki. 1982. "Hybrid Urea Sensor Using Nitrifying Bacteria," *Europ. J. Appl. Microbiol. Biotechnol.*, 14(3):149–154.

16. Zhihong, L., Q. Wenjian, and W. Meng. 1992. "The Preparation of a Spinach Tissue-Based Carbon Paste Microelectrode and Its Performance in Pharmacokinetic Experiments *in vivo*," *Anal. Lett.*, 25(7):1171–1181.

17. Glazier, S. A. and G. A. Rechnitz. 1989. "Construction and Characterization of Beet Stem Based Biosensor for Oxalate," *Anal. Lett.*, 22(15):2929–2948.

18. Wang, J., and A. Brennsteiner. 1988. "Miniature Tissue Based Voltammetric Bioelectrodes," *Anal. Lett.*, 21(10):1773–1783.

19. Wang, J., and M. Shan Lin. 1988. "Mixed Plant Tissue-Carbon Paste Electrode," *Anal. Chem.*, 60(15):1545–1548.

20. Grobler, S. L. and C. W. van Wyg. 1980. "Potentiometric Determination of D(+) Glucose, D(+)Mannose or D(−)Fructose in a Mixture of Hexoses and Pentoses, by Using *Streptococcus mutans* Fermentation," *Talanta*, 27(7):602–604.

21. Karube, I., T. Matsunaga, N. Teraoka, and S. Suzuki. 1980. "Microbioassay of Phenylalanine in Blood Sera with a Lactate Electrode," *Anal. Chim. Acta*, 119: 271–276.

22. Karube, I., T. Okada, and S. Suzuki. 1982. "A Methane Gas Sensor Based on Oxidizing Bacteria," *Anal. Chim. Acta*, 135(1):61–67.

23. Matsunaga, T., I. Karube, and S. Suzuki. 1978. "Electrochemical Microbioassay of Vitamin B_1," *Anal. Chim. Acta*, 98(1):25–30.

24. Simpson, D. L. and R. K. Kobos. 1982. "Microbial Assay of Tetracycline with a Potentiometric CO_2 Gas Sensor," *Anal. Lett.*, 15(B 16):1345–1359.

25. Faria de, L. C., C. Pasquini, and C. de Oliveira Neto. 1991. "Determination of Urea in Serum by Using Naturally Immobilized Urease in a Flow Injection Conductometric System," *Analyst*, 116(4):357–360.

26. Karube, I., S. Mitsuda, T. Matsunaga, and S. Suzuki. 1977. "A Rapid Method for Estimation of BOD by Using Immobilized Microbial Cells," *J. Ferment. Technol.*, 55(3): 243–248.

27. Mattiasson, B., P. O. Larsson, and K. Mosbach. 1977. "The Microbe Thermistor," *Nature*, 268(8):519–520.

28. Kitagawa, Y., E. Tamiya, and I. Karube. 1987. "Microbial-FET Alcohol Sensor," *Anal. Lett.*, 20(1):81–96.

29. Reshetilov, A. N., M. V. Donova, and K. A. Koshcheenko. 1992. "Immobilized Cells of *Gluconobacter oxydans* as a Receptor Element of a Glucose Sensor," *Prikl. Biokhim. Mikrobiol.*, 28(4):518–524 (in Russian).

30. Korpan, Y. I., A. P. Soldatkin, N. F. Starodub, A. V. El'skaya, M. V. Gonchar, A. A. Sibirny, and A. A. Shul'ga. 1993. "Methylotrophic Yeast Microbiosensor Based on Ion-Selective Field Effect Transistors for Methanol and Ethanol Determination," *Anal. Chim. Acta*, 271(2):203–208.

31. Korpan, Y. I., M. V. Gonchar, N. F. Starodub, A. A. Sibirny, and A. V. El'skaya. 1993. "A Cell Biosensor Specific for Formaldehyde Based on pH-Sensitive Transistors Coupled to Methylotrophic Yeast Cells with Genetically Adjusted Metabolism," *Anal. Biochem.*, 215(2):216–222.

32. Arnold, M. A. and G. A. Rechnitz. 1981. "Selectivity Enhancement of a Tissue-Based Adenosine-Sensing Membrane Electrode," *Anal. Chem.*, 53(3):515–518.

33. Hikuma, M., H. Obana, T. Yasuda, I. Karube, and S. Suzuki. 1980. "A Potentiometric Microbial Sensor Based on Immobilized *Escherichia coli* for Glutamic Acid," *Anal. Chim. Acta.*, 116(1):61–67.

34. Kuriyama, S. and G. A. Rechnitz. 1981. "Plant-Tissue Based Bioselective Membrane Electrode for Glutamate," *Anal. Chim. Acta,* 131:91–96.

35. Matsumoto, K., H. Seijo, and T. Watanabe. 1979. "Immobilized Whole Cell-Based Flow-Type Sensor for Cephalosporines," *Anal. Chim. Acta,* 105:429–432.

36. Kobos, R. K., D. J. Rice, and D. S. Flournoy. 1979. "Bacterial Membrane Electrode for the Determination of Nitrate," *Anal. Chem.*, 51(8):1122–1125.

37. Walters, R. R., B. E. Moriarty, and R. P. Buck. 1980. "*Pseudomonas* Bacterial Electrode for Determination of L-Histidine," *Anal. Chem.*, 52(11):1680–1684.

38. Walters, R. R., P. R. Johnson, and R. P. Buck. 1980. "Histidine Ammonia-Lyase Enzyme Electrode for Determination of L-Histidine," *Anal. Chem.*, 52(11):1684–1690.

39. Renneberg, R., K. Riedel, P. Liebs, and F. Scheller. 1984. "Microbial and Hybrid Sensors for Determination of α-Amylase Activity," *Anal. Lett.*, 17(B 5):349–358.

40. Riedel, K., R. Renneberg, R. Kleine, M. Krüger, and F. Scheller. 1988. "A Microbial Sensor for Peptides," *Appl. Microbiol. Biotechnol.*, 28:272–275.

41. Neujahr, H. Y. and K. G. Kjellén. 1979. "Bioprobe Electrode for Phenol," *Biotechnol. Bioeng.*, 21(4):671–678.

42. Macholán, L. and B. Chmelíková. 1986. "Plant Tissue-Based Membrane Biosensor for L-Ascorbic acid, "*Anal. Chim. Acta,* 185:187–193.

43. Ikeda, T., K. Matsuyama, D. Kobayashi, and F. Matsushita. 1992. "Whole-Cell Enzyme Electrodes Based on Mediated Bioelectrocatalysis," *Biosci. Biotech. Biochem.*, 56(8):1359–1360.

44. Pascual, C., R. Pascual, and A. Kotyk. 1982. "Use of Permeabilized Yeast Cells for the Determination of Ethanol and Alcohol Dehydrogenase Assay," *Anal. Biochem.*, 123:205–207.

45. Racek, J. and J. Musil. 1987. "Biosensor for Lactate Determination in Biological Fluids. 1. Construction and Properties of the Biosensor," *Clin. Chim. Acta,* 162(2): 129–139.

46. Vincké, B. J., M. J. Devleeschouwer, and G. J. Patriarche. 1985. "Electrodes potentiometriques et amperometriques a levures permeabilises: determination du L-lactate," *Anal. Lett.*, 18(B 5):593–609.

47. Kulys, J. and Kadziauskiene. 1978. "Bioelectrocatalysis. Lactate-Oxidizing Electrode," *Dokl. Akad. Nauk SSSR,* 239(3):636–639 (in Russian).

48. Karube, I., S. Mitsuda, and S. Suzuki. 1979. "Glucose Sensor Using Immobilized Whole Cells of *Pseudomonas fluorescens*," *Europ. J. Appl. Microbiol. Biotechnol.*, 7: 343–350.

49. Mascini, M. and A. Memoli. 1986. "Comparison of Microbial Sensors Based of Amperometric and Potentiometric Electrodes," *Anal. Chim. Acta,* 182:113–122.

50. Riedel, K., R. Renneberg, and F. Scheller. 1990. "Adaptable Microbial Sensors," *Anal. Lett.*, 23(5):757–770.

51. Hikuma, M., T. Kubo, T. Yasuda, I. Karube, and S. Suzuki. 1979. "Microbial Electrode Sensor for Alcohols," *Biotechnol. Bioeng.*, 21(10):1845–1853.

52. Karube, I., S. Suzuki, T. Okada, and M. Hikuma. 1980. "Microbial Sensors for Volatile Compounds," *Biochimie (Paris)*, 62(8–9):567–573.

53. Hikuma, M., T. Kubo, and T. Yasuda. 1979. "Amperometric Determination of Acetic Acid with Immobilized *Trichosporon brassicae*," *Anal. Chim. Acta*, 109(1):33–38.

54. Hikuma, M., H. Suzuki, T. Yasuda, I. Karube, and S. Suzuki. 1979. "Amperometric Estimation of BOD by Using Living Immobilized Yeasts," *Europ. J. Appl. Microbiol. Biotechnol.*, 8:289–297.

55. Karube, I., T. Matsunaga, S. Mitsuda, and S. Suzuki. 1977. "Microbial Electrode BOD Sensors," *Biotechnol. Bioeng.*, 19:1535–1547.

56. Karube, I., Yokoyama, K. Sode, and E. Tamiya. 1989. "Microbial BOD Sensors Utilizing Thermophillic Bacteria," *Anal. Lett.*, 22(4):791–801.

57. Riedel, K., R. Renneberg, M. Kühn, and F. Scheller. 1988. "A Fast Estimation of Biochemical Oxygen Demand Using Microbial Sensors," *Appl. Microbiol. Biotechnol.*, 28:316–318.

58. Strand, S. E. and D. A. Carlson. 1984. "Rapid BOD Measurement for Municipal Wastewater Samples Using a Biofilm Electrode," *J. Water Pollut. Control. Fed.*, 56(5):464–467.

59. Zhang, X., Z. Jian, and Z. Wanf. 1986. "Microbial Sensor for the BOD Estimation," *Huanjing Kexue Xuebao*, 6(2):184–192 (in Chinese, cited in *Chem. Abstracts*, 1986, 105, 158286).

60. Mattiasson, B., P.-O. Larsson, L. Lindahl, and P. Sahlin. 1982. "Vitamin Analysis with Use of a Yeast Electrode," *Enzyme Microb. Technol.*, 4:153–157.

61. Matsunaga, T., I. Karube, T. Nakahara, and S. Suzuki. 1981. "Amperometric Determination of Viable Cell Numbers Based on Sensing Microbial Respiration," *Europ. J. Appl. Microbiol. Biotechnol.*, 12(1):97–101.

62. Kingdon, C. F. M. 1985. "An Aminoglycoside Biosensor Incorporating Free or Immobilized Bacterial Cells," *Appl. Microbiol. Biotechnol.*, 22(3):165–168.

63. Simpson, D. L. and R. K. Kobos. 1983. "Potentiometric Microbial Assay of Gentamicin, Streptomycin, and Neomycin with a Carbon Dioxide Gas-Sensing Electrode," *Anal. Chem.*, 55:1974–1977.

64. Karube, I., T. Matsunaga, and S. Suzuki. 1979. "Microbioassay of Nystatin with a Yeast Electrode," *Anal. Chim. Acta*, 109(1):39–44.

65. Mascini, M. 1987. "Electrochemical Biosensors for Determination of Nystatin Activity," *Anal. Chim. Acta*, 200:237–244.

66. Karube, I., T. Matsunaga, T. Nakahara, S. Suzuki, and T. Kada. 1981. "Preliminary Screening of Mutagens with a Microbial Sensor," *Anal. Chem.*, 53(7):1024–1026.

67. Riedel, K., P. Liebs, R. Renneberg, and F. Scheller. 1988. "Characterization of the Physiological State of Microorganisms Using the Respiration Electrode," *Anal. Lett.*, 21(8):1305–1322.

68. Hammond, S. M., P. A. Lambert, and B. N. Kliger. 1974. "The Mode of Action of Polyene Antibiotics; Induced Potassium Leakage in *Candida albicans*," *J. Gen. Microbiol.*, 81:325–330.

69. Gale, E. F. 1974. "The Release of Potassium Ions from *Candida albicans* in the Presence of Polyene Antibiotics," *J. Gen. Microbiol.*, 80:451–465.

70. Cosgrove, R. F. 1979. "A Rubidium Ion-Selective Electrode for the Assay of Polyene Antibiotics," *Anal. Chim. Acta*, 105:77–81.

71. D'Orazio, P., M. E. Meyerhoff, and G. A. Rechnitz. 1978. "Membrane Electrode Measurement of Lysozyme Enzyme Using Living Bacterial Cells," *Anal. Chem.*, 50(11):1531–1534.

72. Updike, S. and I. Treichel. 1979. "Antidiuretic Hormone Specific Electrode," *Anal. Chem.*, 51(110):1643–1645.

73. Ho, M. Y. K. and G. A. Rechnitz. 1985. "Potentiometric System for Selective Formate Measurement and Improvement of Response Characteristic by Permeation of Cells," *Biotechnol. Bioeng.*, 27(12):1634–1639.

74. Corcoran, C. A. and R. K. Kobos. 1983. "Selectivity Enhancement of a Bacterial Arginine Electrode," *Anal. Lett.*, 16(B 16):1291–1302.

75. Grobler, S. R. and G. A. Rechitz. 1980. "Determination of D(+)Glucose, D(+)Mannose, D(+)Galactose or D(−)Fructose in a Mixture of Hexoses and Pentoses by Use of Dental Plaque Coupled with a Glass Electrode," *Talanta*, 27(3):283–285.

76. Kulys, J., K. Kadziauskiene, and R. A. Vidziunaite. 1979. "Lactate Oxidation by the Cells of *Hansenula anomala*," *Mikrobiologiya*, 48(4):639–644 (in Russian).

77. Rechnitz, G. A., R. K. Kobos, S. J. Riechel, and C. R. Gebauer. 1977. "A Bio-Selective Membrane Electrode Prepared with Living Bacterial Cells," *Anal. Chim. Acta*, 94(2):357–365.

78. Wollenberger, U., F. Scheller, and P. Atrat. 1980. "Microbial Membrane Electrode for the Determination of Cholesterol," *Anal. Lett.*, 13(B 10):825–836.

79. Schär, H.-P. and O. Ghisalba. 1985. "*Hyphomicrobium* Bacterial Electrode for Determination of Monomethyl Sulfate," *Biotechnol. Bioeng.*, 27:897–901.

80. DiPaolantonio, C. L., M. A. Arnold, and G. A. Rechnitz. 1981. "Serine Selective Membrane Probe Based on Immobilized Anaerobic Bacteria and a Potentiometric Gas Sensor," *Anal. Chim. Acta*, 128:121–127.

81. DiPaolantonio, C. L. and G. A. Rechnitz. 1982. "Induced Bacterial Electrode for the Potentiometric Measurement of Tyrosine," *Anal. Chim. Acta*, 141(1):1–13.

82. DiPaolantonio, C. L. and G. A. Rechnitz. 1983. "Stabilized Bacteria-Based Potentiometric Electrode for Pyruvate," *Anal. Chim. Acta*, 148:1–12.

83. Ihn, G. S. and I. T. Kim. 1989. "Preparation and Comparison of *Proteus vulgaris* and *Proteus mirabilis* Bacterial Electrodes for the Determination of D,L-Phenylalanine," *Bioelectrochem. Bioenerg.*, 21(3):223–232.

84. Ihn, G. S., S. T. Woo, M. J. Sohn, and R. P. Buck. 1989. "Preparation of the *Proteus mirabilis* Bacterial Electrode for the Determination of Urea and Its Clinical Applications," *Anal. Lett.*, 22(1):1–15.

85. Jensen, M. A. and G. A. Rechnitz. 1978. "Bacterial Membrane Electrode for L-Cysteine," *Anal. Chim. Acta*, 101:125–130.

86. Kobos, R. K. and H. A. Pyon. 1981. "Application of Microbial Cells as Multistep Catalyst in Potentiometric Biosensing Electrodes," *Biotechnol. Bioeng.*, 23:627–633.

87. Kobos, R. K. and G. A. Rechnitz. 1977. "Regenerable Bacterial Membrane Electrode for L-Aspartate," *Anal. Lett.*, 10(B 10):751–758.

88. Rechnitz, G. A., T. L. Riechel, R. K. Kobos, and M. E. Meyerhoff. 1984. "Gluta-

mine-Selective Membrane Electrode That Uses Bacterial Cells," *Science*, 199:440–441.

89. Hikuma, M., T. Kubo, and T. Yasuda. 1980. "Ammonia Electrode with Immobilized Nitrifying Bacteria," *Anal. Chem.*, 52(7):1020–1024.

90. Kingdon, C. F. M. 1985. "Biosensor Design: Microbial Loading Capacity of Acetylcellulose Membranes," *Appl. Microbiol. Biotechnol.*, 21(3/4):176–179.

91. Linders, C. R., B. J. Vincké, M. J. Devleeschouwer, and G. J. Patriarche. 1985. "Determinations du tryptophane à l'aide d'electrodes bacteriennes et enzymatiques," *J. Pharm. Belg.*, 40(1) 19–26.

92. Okada, T., I. Karube, and S. Suzuki. 1981. "Microbial Sensor System Which Uses *Methylomonas sp.* for the Determination of Methane," *Europ. J. Appl. Microbiol. Biotechnol.*, 12:102–106.

93. Okada, T., I. Karube, and S. Suzuki. 1983. "NO₂ Sensor Which Uses Immobilized Nitrite Oxidizing Bacteria," *Biotechnol. Bioeng.*, 25:1641–1651.

94. Vincké, B. J., M. J. Devleeschouwer, and G. J. Patriarche. 1983. "Contribution au developpement d'un nouveau modele d'electrode: l'electrode bacterienne," *Anal. Lett.*, 16(B 9):673–684.

95. Vincké, B. J., M. J. Devleeschouwer, and G. J. Patriarche. 1983. "Dosage de l'asparagine à l'aide d'une électrode bacterienne," *J. Pharm. Belg.*, 38(4):225–229.

96. Vincké, B. J., M. J. Devleeschouwer, and G. J. Patriarche. 1985. "Electrode bacterienne en vue de l'utilisation analytique du metabolisme oxydatif du l'tryptophane de *Pseudomonas fluorescens*," *J. Pharm. Belg.*, 40(6):357–365.

97. Matsunaga, T., I. Karube, and S. Suzuki. 1978. "Rapid Determination of Nicotinic Acid by Immobilized *Lactobacillus arabinosus*," *Anal. Chim. Acta*, 99(2):233–239.

98. Hikuma, M., H. Matsuoka, M. Kawarai, and I. Karube. 1992. "Use of Microbial Electrodes for Observation of Microbial Nitrogen Elimination Process," *Biotechnol. Bioeng.*, 40(1):130–136.

99. Burstein, C., E. Adamowicz, K. Boucherit, C. Rabouille, and J.-L. Romette. 1986. "Immobilized Respiratory Chain Activities from *Escherichia coli* Utilized to Measure D- and L-Lactate, Succinate, L-Malate, 3-Glycerophosphate, Pyruvate, or NAD(P)H," *Appl. Biochem. Biotechnol.*, 12(1):1–16.

100. Park, J. K. and H. S. Kim. 1990. A New Biosensor for Specific Determination of Glucose or Fructose Using an Oxidoreductase of *Zymomonas mobilis*," *Biotechnol. Bioeng.*, 36(7):744–749.

101. Racek, J. 1991. "A Yeast Biosensor for Glucose Determination," *Appl. Microbiol. Biotechnol.*, 34(4):473–477.

102. Mandl, M. and L. Macholán. 1990. "Biosensor for the Determination of Iron(II, III) Based on Immobilized Cells of *Thiobacillus ferrooxidans*," *Folia Microbiol.*, 35(4):363–367.

103. Arnold, M. A. and G. A. Rechnitz. 1982. "Optimization of a Tissue-Based Membrane Electrode for Guanine," *Anal. Chem.*, 54(4):777–782.

104. Schubert, F., U. Wollenberger, and F. Scheller. 1983. "Plant Tissue-Based Amperometric Tyrosine Electrode," *Biotechnol. Lett.*, 5(4):239–242.

105. Smit, N. and G. A. Rechnitz. 1984. "Leaf Based Biocatalytic Membrane Electrodes," *Biotechnol. Lett.*, 6(4):209–214.

106. Arnold, M. A. and G. A. Rechnitz. 1980. "Determination of Glutamine in Cerebrospinal Fluid with a Tissue-Based Membrane Electrode," *Anal. Chim. Acta*, 113(2):351–354.

107. Arnold, M. A. and G. A. Rechnitz. 1981. "Tissue-Based Membrane Electrode with High Biocatalytic Activity for Measurement of Adenosine 5'-Monophosphate," *Anal. Chem.*, 53(12):1837–1842.

108. Kuriyama, S., M. A. Arnold, and G. A. Rechnitz. 1983. "Improved Membrane Electrode Using Plant Tissue as Biocatalyst," *J. Membr. Sci.*, 12:269–278.

109. Mascini, M. and G. A. Rechnitz. 1980. "Tissue- and Bacteria-Loaded Tubular Reactors for the Automatic Determination of Glutamine," *Anal. Chim. Acta*, 116(1):169–173.

110. Ma, Y. L. and G. A. Rechnitz. "Porcine Kidney Based Membrane Electrode for Glucosamine-6-phosphate," *Anal. Lett.*, 18(B 13):1635–1646.

111. Mascini, M., M. Iannello, and G. Palleschi. 1982. "A Liver Tissue-Based Electrochemical Sensor for Hydrogen Peroxide," *Anal. Chim. Acta*, 138:65–69.

112. Park, J.-K., H.-S. Ro, and H.-S. Kim. 1991. "A New Biosensor for Specific Determination of Sucrose Using an Oxidoreductase of *Zymomonas mobilis* and Invertase," *Biotechnol. Bioeng.*, 38(3):217–223.

113. Riechel, T. L. and G. A. Rechnitz. 1978. "Hybrid Bacterial and Enzyme Membrane Electrode with Nicotinamide Adenine Dinucleotide Response," *J. Membr. Sci.*, 4:243–250.

114. Linders, C. E., B. J. Vincke, and G. J. Patriarche. 1985. "Electrode hybride pour la determination de phosphates et de polyphosphates. Application aux problemes lies a l'environement," *Anal. Lett.*, 18(B 17):2195–2208.

115. Schubert, F., R. Renneberg, F. W. Scheller, and L. Kirstein. 1984. "Plant Tissue Hybrid Electrode for Determination of Phosphate and Fluoride," *Anal. Chem.*, 56(9): 1677–1682.

116. Svorc, J., S. Miertus, and A. Barlíková. 1990. "Hybrid Biosensor for the Determination of Lactose," *Anal. Chem.*, 62(15):1628–1630.

117. Hartmeier, W. 1985. "Immobilisierte Biokatalysatoren—auf dem Weg zur zweiten Generation," *Naturwissenschaften*, 72:310–314.

118. Campanella, L., M. Cordatore, F. Mazzei, and M. Tomassetti. 1990. "Determination of Inorganic Phosphate in Drug Formulations and Biological Fluids Using a Plant Tissue Electrode," *J. Pharmaceut. Biomed. Anal.*, 8(8–12):711–716.

119. Fonong, T. 1986. "Comparative Study of Potentiometric and Amperometric Tissue-Based Electrodes for Oxalate," *Anal. Chim. Acta*, 186:301–305.

120. Grobler, S. R., N. Basseon, and C. W. van Wyk. 1982. "Bacterial Electrode for L-Arginine," *Talanta*, 29(1):49–51.

121. Kulys, J. J. 1981. "The Development of New Analytical Systems Based on Biocatalysts," *Anal. Lett.*, 14(B 6):377–397.

122. Suzuki, M., S. Lee, K. Fujii, I. Arikawa, I. Kubo, T. Kanagawa, E. Mikami, and I. Karube. 1992. "Determination of Sulfite Ion by Using Microbial Sensor," *Anal. Lett.*, 25(6):973–982.

123. Uchiyama, S. and G. A. Rechnitz. 1987. "Biosensor Using Flower Petal Structures," *J. Electroanal. Chem.* 222:343–346.

124. Arnold, M. A. and S. A. Glazier. 1984. "Jack Bean Meal as Biocatalyst for Urea Biosensors," *Biotechnol. Lett.*, 6(6):313–318.

125. Hikuma, M., H. Obana, T. Yasuda, I. Karube, and S. Suzuki. 1980. "Amperometric Determination of Total Assimilable Sugars in Fermentation Broths with Use of Immobilized Whole Cells," *Enzyme Microb. Technol.*, 2:234–238.

126. Lowry, J. P. and R. D. O'Neill. 1992. "Homogeneous Mechanism of Ascorbic Acid In-

terference in Hydrogen Peroxide Detection at Enzyme-Modified Electrodes," *Anal. Chem.*, 64(4):453-456 (letter).

127. Montalvo, J. and G. G. Guilbault. 1969. "Sensitized Cation Selective Electrode," *Anal. Chem.*, 41(1):1897-1899.

128. Wollenberger, U., F. Scheller, and P. Atrat. 1980. "Microbial Membrane Electrode for Steroid Assay," *Anal. Lett.*, 13(B 13):1201-1210.

129. Ukeda, H., G. Wagner, U. Bilitewski, and R. D. Schmid. 1992. "Flow Injection Analysis of Short-Chain Fatty Acids in Milk Based on a Microbial Electrode," *J. Agr. Food. Chem.*, 40(11):2324-2327.

130. Uchiyama, S., M. Tamata, Y. Tofuku, and S. Suzuki. 1988. "A Catechol Electrode Based on Spinach Leaves," *Anal. Chim. Acta*, 208:287-290.

131. Navaratne, A., M. S. Lin, and G. A. Rechnitz. 1990. "Eggplant Based Bioamperometric Sensor for the Detection of Catechol," *Anal. Chim. Acta*, 237:107-113.

132. Racek, J. and J. Musil. 1987. "Biosensor for Lactate Determination in Biological Fluids. 2. Interference Studies," *Clin. Chim. Acta*, 167(1):59-65.

133. Kawashima, T., K. Tomida, N. Tominaga, T. Kobayashi, and H. Onishi. 1984. "A Microbial Sensor for Uric Acid," *Chem. Lett. (Chem. Soc. Japan)*, 5:653-656.

134. Tsuchida, T., and K. Yoda. 1983. "Multi-Enzyme Membrane Electrodes for Determination of Creatinine and Creatine in Serum," *Clin. Chem.*, 29(1):51-55.

135. Karube, I., T. Nakahara, T. Matsunaga, and S. Suzuki. 1982. "*Salmonella* Electrode for Screening Mutagens," *Anal. Chem.*, 54(11):1725-1727.

136. Karube, I. and S. Suzuki. 1984. "Amperometric and Potentiometric Determinations with Immobilized Enzymes and Microorganisms," *Ion-Selective Electrode Rev.*, 6(1): 15-58.

137. Rosario, S. A., G. S. Cha, M. E. Meyerhoff, and M. Trojanowicz. 1990. "Use of Ionomer Membranes to Enhance the Selectivity of Electrode-Based Biosensors in Flow-Injection Analysis," *Anal. Chem.*, 62(15):2418-2424.

138. Nagy, G., M. E. Rice, and R. N. Adams. 1982. "A New Type of Enzyme Electrode: the Ascorbic Acid Eliminator Electrode," *Life Sci.*, 31(23):2611-2616.

139. Maidan, R. and A. Heller. 1992. "Elimination of Electrooxidizable Interferant-Produced Currents in Amperometric Biosensors," *Anal. Chem.*, 64(23):2889-2896.

140. Tsuchida, T. and K. Yoda. 1981. "Immobilization of D-Glucose Oxidase onto a Hydrogen Peroxide Permselective Membrane and Application for an Enzyme Electrode," *Enzyme Microb. Technol.*, 3:326-330.

141. Renneberg, R., F. Scheller, K. Riedel, E. Litschko, and M. Richter. 1983. "Development of Anti-Interference Enzyme Layer for α-Amylase Measurements in Glucose Containing Samples," *Anal. Lett.*, 16(B 12):877-890.

142. Barlíková, A., J. Svorc, and S. Miertus. 1991. "Hybrid Biosensor for the Determination of Sucrose," *Anal. Chim. Acta*, 242:83-87.

143. Suzuki, H., E. Tamiya, and I. Karube. 1987. "An Amperometric Sensor for Carbon Dioxide Based on Immobilized Bacteria Utilizing Carbon Dioxide," *Anal. Chim. Acta*, 199:85-91.

144. Riedel, K. and F. Scheller. 1987. "Inhibitor-Treated Microbial Sensor for the Selective Determination of Glutamic Acid," *Analyst*, 112(3):341-342.

145. Simonian, A. L., E. I. Rainina, V. I. Lozinsky, I. E. Badalian, G. E. Khachatrian, S. Sh. Tatikian, T. A. Makhlis, and S. D. Varfolomeyev. 1992. "A Biosensor for L-Proline Determination by Use of Immobilized Microbial Cells," *Appl. Biochem. Biotechnol.*, 26(3):199-210.

146. Somlo, M. 1965. "Induction des lactico-cytochrome *c* reductases (D- at L-) de la levure aerobic par les lactates (D- et L-)," *Biochim. Biophys. Acta,* 97(1):183–201.

147. Renneberg, R., K. Riedel, and F. Scheller. 1985. "Microbial Sensor for Aspartame," *Appl. Microbiol. Biotechnol.,* 21(3/4):180–181.

148. Karube, I., S. Sogabe, T. Matsunaga, and S. Suzuki. 1983. "Sulfite Ions Sensor with Use of Immobilized Organelle," *Eur. J. Appl. Microbiol. Biotechnol.,* 17:216–220.

149. Schubert, F., F. Scheller, and D. Kirstein. 1982. "Microsomal Electrodes for Reduced Nicotinamide Adenine Dinucleotide and Its Phosphate, Glucose-6-phosphate and Ascorbate," *Anal. Chim. Acta,* 141:15–21.

150. Corcoran, C. A. and R. K. Kobos. 1987. "Selectivity Enhancement of an *Escherichia coli* Bacterial Electrode Using Enzyme and Transport Inhibitors," *Biotechnol. Bioeng.,* 30(9):565–570.

151. Kulys, J. and K. Kadziauskiene. 1980. "Yeast BOD Sensor," *Biotechnol. Bioeng.,* 22:221–226.

152. Svorc, J., K. Katrlík, and S. Miertus. 1992. "Whole Cell *Aspergillus niger* Biosensor for Determination of Glucose," *Trends Electrochem. Biosensors,* UNIDO ICS Trieste, Italy.

153. Kluys, J., V. Laurinavichus, M. Pesliakiene, and V. Gureviciene. 1983. "The Determination of Glucose, Hypoxanthine and Uric Acid with Use of Bi-Enzyme Amperometric Electrodes," *Anal. Chim. Acta,* 148:13–18.

154. Sidwell, J. S. and G. A. Rechnitz. 1986. "'Bananatrode'—An Electrochemical Biosensor for Dopamine," *Biotechnol. Lett.,* 7(6):419–422.

155. Mascini, M. and G. Palleschi. 1983. "A Tissue-Based Electrode for Peroxidase Assay: Preliminary Results in Hormone Determination by EIA," *Anal. Lett.,* 16(B 14):1053–1066.

156. Racek, J. and R. Petr. 1990. "Possibilities of Using Catalase Erythrocyte Biosensor for Hydrogen Peroxide Determination in Enzyme Immunoassay," *Biochem. Clin. Bohemoslov.,* 19(5):455–457 (in Czech).

157. Rechnitz, G. A. and M. Meyerhoff. 1978. "Biochemical Electrodes Uses Tissue Slices," *Chem. Eng. News,* 56(41):16.

158. Suzuki, H., E. Tamiya, I. Karube, and T. Oshima. 1988. "Carbon Dioxide Sensor Using Thermophilic Bacteria," *Anal. Lett.,* 21(8):1323–1336.

159. Vais, H., F. Oancea, A. M. Fagliu, C. Delcea, and D. G. Margineanu. 1985. "Amperometric Electrode for Glucose with Immobilized Bacteria (*Pseudomonas fluorescens*)," *Rev. Roum. Biochim.,* 2(1):57–63.

160. Meyerhoff, M. E. 1980. "Preparation and Response Properties of Selective Bioelectrodes Utilizing Polymer Membrane Electrode-Based Ammonia Gas Sensors," *Anal. Lett.,* 13(B 15):1345–1357.

161. Scheller, F., F. Schubert, D. Pfeiffer, I. Dransfeld, R. Renneberg, U. Wollenberger, K. Riedel, M. Pavlova, M. Kühn, H.-G. Müller, P. Tan, W. Hoffmann, and W. Moritz. 1989. "Research and Development of Biosensors," *Analyst,* 114:653–662.

162. Navaratne, A. and G. A. Rechnitz. 1992. "Improved Plant-Tissue Based Biosensor Using *in vitro* Cultured Tobacco Callus Tissue," *Anal. Chim. Acta,* 257:59–66.

163. Riedel, K., J. Hensel. S. Rothe, B. Neumann, and F. Scheller. 1993. "Microbial Sensors for Determination of Aromatics and Their Chloroderivatives. 2. Determination of Chlorinated Phenols Using a *Rhodococcus*-Containing Biosensor," *App. Microbiol. Biotechnol.,* 38(4):556–559.